SECOND EDITION

Manual of Clinical Hysteroscopy

SECOND EDITION

Manual of Clinical Hysteroscopy

Rafael F. Valle MD

Professor, Department of Obstetrics and Gynecology
Northwestern University Medical School
Chicago, Illinois, USA

Foreword by

John J. Sciarra MD, PhD
Thomas J. Watkins Professor and Chair
Department of Obstetrics and Gynecology
Northwestern University Medical School
Chicago, Illinois, USA

Taylor & Francis
Taylor & Francis Group

LONDON AND NEW YORK

A PARTHENON BOOK

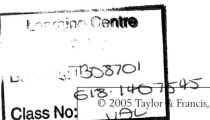
© 2005 Taylor & Francis, an imprint of the Taylor & Francis Group

First published in the United Kingdom in 2005
by Taylor & Francis,
an imprint of the Taylor & Francis Group,
2 Park Square, Milton Park
Abingdon, Oxon OX14 4RN, UK

Tel.: +44 (0) 1235 828600
Fax.: +44 (0) 1235 829000
Website: www.tandf.co.uk

British Library Cataloguing in Publication Data

Data available on application

Library of Congress Cataloging-in-Publication Data

Data available on application

ISBN 1-84214-259-3

Distributed in North and South America by

Taylor & Francis
2000 NW Corporate Blvd
Boca Raton, FL 33431, USA

Within Continental USA
Tel.: 800 272 7737; Fax.: 800 374 3401
Outside Continental USA
Tel.: 561 994 0555; Fax.: 561 361 6018
E-mail: orders@crcpress.com

Distributed in the rest of the world by
Thomson Publishing Services
Cheriton House
North Way
Andover, Hampshire SP10 5BE, UK
Tel.: +44 (0) 1264 332424
E-mail: salesorder.tandf@thomsonpublishingservices.co.uk

Composition by Parthenon Publishing
Printed and bound by T.G. Hostench S.A., Spain

Contents

Dedication

*To my teachers, my family and my patients,
who have kept me focused towards achieving my
intended objective*

Preface to second edition

The first edition of *A Manual of Clinical Hysteroscopy* was completed in 1995 and published in 1997. Over the following 8 years, several innovations, while not fundamental, have occurred in hysteroscopy. Office hysteroscopy has been simplified with the use of small-caliber, continuous-flow hysteroscopes provided with enhanced high-resolution lenses and 5-French operative channels that permit not only good visualization but also the performance of certain operative procedures in the office setting. The standard operative hysteroscopes have also been improved, with continuous-flow systems and sturdier 7-French operative instruments. The resectoscopes have been refined, providing easier maneuverability and applications in the uterine cavity; at the same time, the effect of continuous cleansing of the uterine cavity has been improved. Bipolar-like resectoscopes now permit the use of electrolyte-containing fluids, encouraging physicians to use these methods more frequently. Finally, the applications of hysteroscopy have been better defined and expanded to include sterilization, and more gynecologists have been trained in performing hysteroscopic procedures.

In this second edition, I have tried to keep the original qualities of the manual, such as easiness in reading, concise descriptions and practical guidelines for the performance of diagnostic and operative hysteroscopy. I have resisted the temptation to pack the book with esoteric considerations not applicable in the clinical setting, but rather, have maintained its didactic core and practicality. Some changes have been implemented to keep up with the innovations that have occurred. The intrauterine pictures have been printed in color to enhance their didactic message and the references updated, but only with those that I consider important to the message conveyed in each chapter.

I hope this second edition of the *Manual of Clinical Hysteroscopy* will meet your needs and will also increase interest in hysteroscopy and hysteroscopic surgery for practicing gynecologists, resulting in improved care for their patients.

I would like to thank my contributors for their attentive revision and update of their respective chapters, and also, Taylor & Francis Medical Books for the prompt and timely review and publication of the manuscript.

Rafael F. Valle MD
Chicago

Preface to first edition

As a self-taught hysteroscopist, over the years I have faced the many inconveniences and handicaps that usually accompany a new technique. In 1972, as a neophyte hysteroscopist, I paid a visit to Dr Rodolfo Quinones in Mexico City to observe his technique of hysteroscopy using low-viscosity fluids. Following this visit, I adapted a similar technique, using polyethylene catheters to convert the hysteroscope into a continuous-flow system. In addition, I modified the delivery system by using plastic containers that could be converted, in systems using positive pressure, by external pressure cuffs. These minor modifications assisted me in the application of low-viscosity fluids for intrauterine distention as an alternative to CO_2 gas and high-viscosity dextrans, and permitted not only distention, but also intermittent washings, particularly during operative procedures.

In 1976, as hysteroscopic clinical applications became more extensive, I began to offer a hysteroscopy workshop to gynecologists on a yearly basis. As the gynecological resectoscope and lasers were introduced, these methods were also incorporated into our clinical practice. Thus, after nearly a quarter of a century of experience in adapting methods, instrumentation and expanding clinical applications, I was rewarded with an efficient, relatively easy and effective hysteroscopy program that many physicians have subsequently adapted for themselves.

Being aware of the need for a concise, practical book on hysteroscopy with a unified philosophy, I have brought together in this volume a didactic core of diagnostic and operative hysteroscopy as a practical and concise reference volume. This manual is aimed at residents, fellows and practicing gynecologists with an interest in hysteroscopy. Although there are selected references for each chapter, it was not my intention to provide an encyclopedic bibliography.

The illustrations included in this book have been selected to show, in conjunction with the instructive 'how-to' drawings, the normal and abnormal presentations in selected instances as well as the various operative steps in selected procedures to provide the practitioner with a better understanding of the methods used. However, sound clinical medical judgment cannot be replaced by a procedure and, therefore, I have included a discussion of the indications and contraindications of hysteroscopy as well as of the management of complications, with practical guidelines for the prevention of specific complications. I hope the reader will find this to be a practical manual of the rationale and techniques for the optimal performance of various hysteroscopic procedures.

To complete the theme of uterine evaluation, there are also four chapters written by four guest contributors: Dr Alvin Siegler on hysterosalpingography; Dr Leeber Cohen on ultrasonography; Dr Frederick Hoff on computed tomography and magnetic resonance imaging; and Dr Debra Heller on uterine pathology. I am indebted to these experts for their invaluable contributions.

I am also grateful to the many colleagues who have shared their experiences and suggestions with me, in particular, Dr John J. Sciarra who, as Chairman of the Department of Obstetrics and Gynecology at Northwestern University Medical School, as well as my teacher and mentor, has sparked, and consistently encouraged and supported, my interest in hysteroscopy.

Finally, I am grateful to Parthenon Publishing for their invaluable help in making this manual a reality.

In closing, if this book provides a useful aid to physicians who are learning hysteroscopy, reassures those who are already accomplished in the procedure and improves the care provided to patients, then my goal in writing this manual will have been fulfilled.

Rafael F. Valle MD
Chicago

Foreword

Hysteroscopy is a dynamic and essential part of contemporary gynecological practice. *Manual of Clinical Hysteroscopy* by Dr Rafael Valle is a wonderful concise and comprehensive practical text which covers both diagnostic and operative hysteroscopy.

The possibility of visualizing the interior of the uterus has interested physicians for the past 100 years. Hysteroscopy, however, did not become a standard reproducible clinical procedure until the advent of modern instrumentation. This manual is a fully illustrated and well-written presentation of the instruments and techniques that have evolved over the past two decades. The content is designed to serve as both a resource for the physician who is currently using hysteroscopy and also an introductory text for those who are in the process of developing their skills with the technique.

In many ways, this book represents the cumulative experience and career of its author, Dr Valle, who is recognized to be one of the senior international authorities and leaders in the field of hysteroscopy and hysteroscopic surgery. Through his current position as a professor of obstetrics and gynecology at Northwestern University Medical School in Chicago, he has over the years personally taught the skills and techniques of diagnostic hysteroscopy and operative hysteroscopy to a large number of residents and practitioners. With this manual,

we now have available to us the didactic material compiled over his many years of teaching hysteroscopy. The readers of this book, whether they be young physicians, accomplished practitioners or enthusiasts, will all benefit from the practical and useful guidelines developed by this one man who has had over 25 years of clinical experience in this field.

One of the best features of this book is its readability. A further plus is the continuity of presentation, as virtually all of the material has been prepared by the same author, with the exception of the four chapters on the various imaging modalities and pathology written by experts in those fields.

All invasive procedures must be accompanied by appropriate indications. Another strength of this text is its comprehensive presentation of the indications and contraindications for hysteroscopy. Although complications from the procedure are rare, it remains important that the practitioner be aware of the possible complications. Indeed, this book contains an excellent chapter on the subject.

Following a chapter devoted to office hysteroscopy, the reader is led into the exciting field of surgical hysteroscopic therapy. In these chapters, the author presents a clear and conservative portrayal of the value of operative hysteroscopic procedures, drawing from the available evidence as well as his own extensive and practical experience.

Finally, this manual includes some excellent photographs of typical intrauterine pathology and several clarifying diagrams, a number of which were specially prepared for inclusion in this book.

Manual of Clinical Hysteroscopy is an important contribution to the gynecological literature of our time. It presents state-of-the-art information on gynecological endoscopy together with the extensive personal experience of Dr Valle, one of the true pioneers in the field.

I believe this manual will become a classic addition to the libraries of all practicing gynecologists and gynecological surgeons. No one in this field could want a better practical reference guide than this excellent volume.

John J. Sciarra MD PhD
Chicago

1

An introduction to hysteroscopy

Evaluation of the uterine cavity is necessary when abnormal bleeding develops and/or reproduction is impaired. Because the endometrium changes cyclically and continuously under the influence of steroids, its structure and thickness also vary and, when abnormal growth occurs, it is important to rule out those conditions that not only may be the cause of the abnormal bleeding, but may predispose the patient to malignancy. Premalignant and malignant lesions of the endometrium need to be ruled out. Other benign conditions within the uterus, such as endometrial polyps and uterine leiomyomas, may also cause abnormal bleeding and require treatment. Finally, structural uterine developmental anomalies can occur as a result of abnormal embryogenesis, and hysteroscopy provides an excellent method of evaluation and treatment when these conditions impair reproduction.

Traditionally, the uterine cavity has been evaluated with mechanical curettes, forceps, sounds or probes, suction devices and hysterosalpingography. Whereas suction devices are useful in obtaining endometrium for histological evaluation, they may not provide accurate diagnosis of endometrial polyps and/or leiomyomas. Blind uterine exploration with curettes or forceps also lacks accuracy in evaluating the endometrial lining.

With the use of small and thin suction devices activated not by pumps, but by small plungers, endometrial evaluation becomes more difficult, particularly if the entire endometrial lining must be evaluated. These devices are most useful when the endometrium is sampled to determine the stage of maturation in infertility evaluation. When used for evaluation of abnormal uterine bleeding, however, they may not provide adequate tissue for a complete histological evaluation of the endometrial lining. Hysterosalpingography under fluoroscopic view allows evaluation of the symmetry of the uterine cavity and rules out space-occupying lesions such as polyps and/or myomas. In addition, this method provides evaluation of the Fallopian tubes, revealing their caliber, distal epithelial folds and patency. Whereas hysterosalpingography is most valuable when normal findings are obtained, additional evaluation may be necessary – should abnormal findings be encountered – to rule out false distortions simulating pathology.

Following clinical trials to establish the indications and proper place of hysteroscopy in clinical gynecology, the use of hysteroscopy expanded in the 1980s to the point where, today, it is a well-established method of evaluation and treatment of many conditions of the uterine cavity. Of late, new methods of evaluating the uterus, such as ultrasound particularly with vaginal probes, fluid-enhanced sonography and hysteroscopy, have been introduced.

Sonography allows evaluation of the uterine walls, which is not possible with endoscopic methods. The practitioner is able to rule out the presence of leiomyomas or assess their location, size and number. The endometrial lining can be evaluated and measured, particularly in post-menopausal patients who bleed abnormally.

Fluid-enhanced sonography adds another dimension to the ultrasound examination by adding contrast and permitting better evaluation of intrauterine lesions such as polyps and myomas. Because of this, the technique helps to determine the degree of penetration of these lesions into the myometrial wall, and the intramural and intraluminal components.

Hysteroscopy offers a direct view of the uterine cavity and the possibility of targeted biopsies of suspect areas. Special hysteroscopes can evaluate tissues at various magnifications, from ×20 to ×150, or at nucleocytoplasmic levels.

Recently, microendoscopes with outer diameters <3 mm were introduced to allow easier transcervical introduction and avoid anesthesia. The practical value of these endoscopes is currently being studied.

This manual reviews various aspects of diagnostic and therapeutic hysteroscopy. The current instrumentation required for diagnosis and treatment is described with practical observations regarding their use. The diagnostic and therapeutic applications of hysteroscopy, including its various indications, contraindications and possible complications, are also reviewed. The fundamental steps in the performance of diagnostic and operative hysteroscopy and resectoscopy are described with practical recommendations for simplifying the procedures.

HISTORICAL LANDMARKS IN THE DEVELOPMENT OF HYSTEROSCOPY

The major historical landmarks in the development of hysteroscopy are summarized in Table 1.1. In 1807, Philip Bozzini developed the first known endoscope to view the interior of the uterus and/or urinary bladder (Figure 1.1). In 1853, Antonin Désormeaux presented a model of the first truly workable cystoscope (Figure 1.2) to the French Academy of Medicine. This scope had a reflecting mirror with a central perforation for viewing. However, it was not

Figure 1.1 Bozzini's light conductor, devised in the early 1800s, was a candlelit specular instrument for illumination of body cavities

Table 1.1 Milestones in the development of hysteroscopy

Year	Investigator	Contribution
1807	Bozzini	First endoscope (light conductor)
1869	Pantaleoni	First hysteroscopic examination in living patient
1879	Nitze	Cystoscope with distal illumination
1907	David	First contact hysteroscope
1914	Heineberg	System for irrigating uterine cavity
1925	Rubin	CO_2 for uterine distention
1926	Seymour	Hysteroscope with inflow and outflow channels
1927	Mikulicz-Radecki and Freund	Biopsy-taking capability, cornual electrocoagulation
1928	Gauss	Intrauterine photography
1934	Schroeder	Measurement of intrauterine pressures
1934–1943	Segond	Irrigating system and biopsies
1936	Schack	Identified applications
1942–1970	Norment	Rubber balloon, practical irrigating system, cutting loop, fiberoptics
1953–1978	Mohri and Mohri	Fiberhysteroscope for intrauterine visualization tubaloscopy
1957	Englund *et al.*	Evaluation of abnormal uterine bleeding comparing hysterography and dilatation and curettage with hysteroscopy
1962	Silander	Studied endometrial carcinoma using silastic balloon
1968	Menken	Tubal cannulation, polyvinylpyrrolidone
1970	Edstrom and Fernstrom	32% dextran
1972	Quinones *et al.*	Tubal catheterization applications
1974	Edstrom	Therapeutic applications
1974	Parent *et al.*	Contact hysteroscopy
1978	Neuwirth	Use of resectoscope
1980	Hamou	Microhysteroscope
1981	Goldrath *et al.*	Laser endometrial ablation

until 1869 that Pantaleoni used a modified endoscope in a clinical setting to evaluate the uterine cavity in a postmenopausal patient complaining of abnormal uterine bleeding. Polyps were found and cauterized with silver nitrate, using the endoscope as a guide.

The first practical contact endoscope was introduced by David in 1907. This endoscope had a distal lens that permitted visualization of uterine lesions on contact. No distending medium was necessary and external light was introduced into the uterus by reflection. Heineberg in 1914 and Seymour in 1935 advanced the possibilities of continuous-flow systems to look into the uterus. Practical methods using low-viscosity fluids to distend the uterus were introduced by Norment in 1950, followed in 1958 by the application of the first rudimentary gynecological resectoscope with a loop electrode to remove myomas and polyps. In the late 1960s, Menken developed a special hysteroscope designed for tubal cannulation (Figure 1.3), using a high-viscosity mixture of linear polymers of

Figure 1.2 Désormeaux's first workable endoscope (left), as presented to the French Academy of Medicine in 1853, comprised a jar at the bottom holding alcohol, with a wick that extended into the central part of the instrument (middle). A cutaway view (right) shows that the flame in the central part of the instrument had a reflecting mirror to the right and a lens to the left

Figure 1.3 The hysteroscope devised by Menken in the late 1960s for tubal cannulation

different chain lengths and molecular weights, or polyvinylpyrrolidone, allowing passage of catheters into the tubal ostium.

In 1970, Edstrom and Fernstrom introduced a method of hysteroscopy using a high-viscosity dextran (Hyskon®) that improved visualization and permitted intra-uterine surgery. Lindemann perfected the delivery of CO_2 gas as a distending medium for hysteroscopy, with special machines designed to calibrate the flow and intrauterine pressure produced by the gas. In 1974, the initial therapeutic applications of hysteroscopy were established by Edstrom,

including the division of intra-uterine adhesions, treatment of uterine septa and resection of submucous leiomyomas.

In 1980, a microcolpohysteroscope was introduced by Hamou. This instrument permitted magnification of tissue at different degrees – ×20, ×60 and ×150 – or at nucleocytoplasmic levels. The neodymium : yttrium–aluminum–garnet (Nd : YAG) laser was approved by the US Food and Drug Administration (FDA) as a tool to perform endometrial ablation in 1986, and the resectoscope was approved for gynecological procedures in 1989. In the late 1980s, a high-resolution, high-sensitivity, light video camera was specifically designed for endoscopy.

On November 4, 2002 the ESSURE™ hysteroscopic tubal sterilization method was approved by the FDA for clinical use in the USA.

While the technology continues to develop, the improvements in instrumentation and ancillary equipment have kept pace with the use and applications of hysteroscopy as a diagnostic and therapeutic tool.

SELECTED BIBLIOGRAPHY

Bush RB, Leonhardt H, Bush IM, Lands RR. Dr Bozzini's Lichtleiter. A translation of his original article (1806). *Urology* 1974;3:119

Harrison RM. The development of modern endoscopy. *J Med Primatol* 1976;5:73

Lindemann HJ. Historical aspects of hysteroscopy. *Fertil Steril* 1973;24:230

Norment WB. The hysteroscope. *Am J Obstet Gynecol* 1956;71:426

Pearlman SJ. Bozzini's classical treatise on endoscopy: a translation. *Q Bull Northwest Univ Med School* 1949;23:332

Rathert P, Lutzeyer W, Goddwin WE. Philip Bozzini (1773–1809) and the Lichtleiter. *Urology* 1974;3:113

Valle RF. Hysteroscopy. In Wynn RM, ed. Obstetrics and Gynecology Annual, Vol. 7. New York: *Appleton-Century-Crofts*, 1978: 245–83

Valle RF, Sciarra JJ. Current status of hysteroscopy in gynecologic practice. *Fertil Steril* 1979;32:619

2

General principles and instrumentation

The basic requirements for the performance of hysteroscopy include an endoscope or hysteroscope, media to distend the cavity of the uterus, and an appropriate light source to transmit adequate illumination via fiberoptic cables.

Although the first known endoscope to observe hollow organs, such as the urinary bladder and the uterus, was introduced by Bozzini in 1807, the practical clinical applications of endoscopy to visualize the uterine cavity did not occur until the late 1960s and early 1970s, with the introduction of endoscopes specifically designed to visualize this organ. The most cumbersome impediment to the use of hysteroscopy in a clinical setting was solved with the availability of safe and effective media to distend the uterine cavity. Fiberoptics has greatly improved visualization by illuminating this small cavity that is surrounded by thick muscular layers.

THE HYSTEROSCOPE

There are two types of hysteroscope – rigid and flexible. Modern rigid hysteroscopes are of two kinds – diagnostic and operative.

Diagnostic hysteroscopes

These are in general no larger than 4 mm in outer diameter and permit uterine distention by delivering CO_2 gas (Figure 2.1). Because of their size, these hysteroscopes do not provide an operative channel. The telescope has either a straightforward 0° angle of view or a 30° foreoblique view, which is most commonly used to visualize the uterotubal junctions. There are other diagnostic hysteroscopes with slightly larger outer diameters of 5–6 mm, with distal fenestrations that permit continuous flow when low-viscosity fluids are used to distend the uterus. Although these hysteroscopes may also have small operating channels, only mild conditions can be treated, and biopsies taken with small-caliber forceps are gener-

Figure 2.1 Diagnostic and operative hysteroscope with continous-flow sheaths and 5-Fr operative instrument in place (Storz)

Figure 2.2 Compact hysteroscope (15-Fr diameter) with handle (upper), and 5-Fr semirigid forceps and grasper (middle and lower) (Wolf)

Figure 2.3 ACMI Slimline™ operative hysteroscope. Inset shows ports of continuous-flow system

Figure 2.4 Oval sheaths (4.9×3.9 mm outer diameter) for continuous-flow hysteroscopy (Storz)

ally inadequate for proper histological evaluation (Figures 2.2 and 2.3).

Other diagnostic hysteroscopes may have the capability of magnification, such as the Hamou hysteroscope or microcolpohysteroscope, with an additional offside ocular that can increase the magnification 20-fold for a panoramic view, or to ×60 or ×150 for a contact view. The latter magnification can evaluate tissues at the nucleocytoplasmic level. The instrument can also be used for evaluation of the ectocervix on contact.

With advances in endoscopic technology, new small-caliber hysteroscopes were introduced in the early 1990s that resolved some of the drawbacks previously seen with the original single-flow small-caliber hysteroscopes. One was the introduction of continuous flow to permit not only uterine distention but also continuous washing of the uterine cavity. The second was the introduction of telescopes based on both the rod lens system and fiberoptic technology that permitted these small-diameter telescopes to project efficient light and also improve their resolution. Finally, video cameras were enhanced by the addition of zooming mechanisms that increased the size of the image provided by these small telescopes and focusing in order to observe details of the

Figure 2.5 Close-up view of distal tip of a diagnostic-operative hysteroscope with a continuous-flow outer sheath and semirigid forceps in the operating channel (ACMI)

Figure 2.6 Various operative instruments (5-Fr), from left to right: corkscrew to fix myomas, sharp scissors, blunt scissors, punch-biopsy forceps, spoon-biopsy forceps and grasping forceps (Storz)

Figure 2.7 Vaporizing electrode (Versapoint) that can be used under electrolytic fluids. (a) Twizzle electrode, (b) spring electrodes (GyneCare)

uterine cavity during evaluation. Additionally, an array of mechanical instruments of the 5-French (5-Fr) caliber were designed for operative procedures. Some continuous-flow sheaths have an oval profile (3.9 × 5.9 mm), others are round for operative hysteroscopy with liquid distention medium. The telescopes used vary from 2 to 2.9 mm in diameter (Figures 2.4–2.7).

The flexible diagnostic hysteroscopes, usually 3.5 mm in outer diameter, are excellent alternatives for diagnosis (Figure 2.8). In addition to their distal steerability,

Figure 2.8 Flexible diagnostic hysteroscope (3.5 mm outer diameter) (Fujinon)

Figure 2.9 Operative hysteroscope (7 mm outer diameter) with flexible forceps in place (Storz)

Figure 2.10 Diagnostic–operative hysteroscope with (lower) and without (upper) continuous-flow outer sheath (Wolf)

they have an additional feature that allows the tip to be bent according to need. This can be helpful in markedly anteflexed or retro-flexed uteri in guiding the instrument atraumatically towards the uterine cavity. When pathology such as tumors that distort the symmetry of the uterine cavity or intrauterine adhesions is present, the steerability of this instrument helps in the guided introduction and exploration of the uterus. With these flexible diagnostic hysteroscopes, either CO_2 gas or low-viscosity fluids can be used as distending media.

Figure 2.11 Double-channel operating hysteroscope with ancillary instruments in place (Bryan)

Operative hysteroscopes

These hysteroscopes have telescopes 4 mm in outer diameter and require a larger operative sheath, usually 7–8 mm in outer diameter, and an operative channel to permit 7-Fr instruments, either flexible or semirigid, to be inserted and manipulated (Figure 2.9). Most modern operative hysteroscopes have some type of continuous-flow system to permit washing of the uterine cavity (Figure 2.10), but because this washing effect is not as efficient as that provided by the resectoscope when targeted areas need to be cleansed of blood clots or debris, a polyethylene catheter is inserted in the operating channel to perform this specific function. Recently, outer sheaths with distal fenestrations have been used to permit retrieval and collection of fluid, and continuous lavage of the uterine cavity.

New hysteroscopes with more than one operating channel have been designed to permit not only continuous flow, but addi-

Figure 2.12 Flexible operative hysteroscope (4.9 mm diameter) with flexible forceps in place (Fujinon)

Figure 2.13 Semirigid ancillary hysteroscopic instruments (7-Fr diameter) include, from upper to lower, biopsy forceps, scissors and grasping forceps (Storz)

tional means of surgical manipulation in the uterine cavity. The outer diameter of these instruments can be increased to 8–9 mm, so these instruments require cervical dilatation of 9.5–10 mm (Figure 2.11).

Flexible operative hysteroscopes are also available with an outer diameter of 4.9 mm and an operating channel with an inner diameter of 2.5 mm for instrumentation (Figure 2.12). Flexible operative hysteroscopes permit the introduction of significantly smaller instruments than permitted with rigid instrumentation without significant cervical dilatation, thereby decreasing trauma. Because of their capability for flexing the distal tip, they are excellent alternatives for tubal cannulation, permitting catheters to be placed in the direction of the tubal opening. This is particularly useful in patients with laterally recessed tubal cornual junctions and in those who have T-shaped uterine cavities. Fiberoptic lasers can be guided more easily through flexible hysteroscopes, should they be required for treatment of lesions at the cornua or for laterally placed lesions in the uterine walls such as intrauterine adhesions.

Figure 2.14 Sturdy optical scissors fixed at the distal end of a hysteroscope (Olympus)

ANCILLARY INSTRUMENTS

To perform hysteroscopic surgery, several instruments may be required, such as scissors, grasping forceps, biopsy forceps, catheters and electroprobes. These instruments are usually 7-Fr in diameter and fit snugly in the operating channel. The most commonly used ancillary operative instruments are the semirigid type (Figure 2.13) that can be bent somewhat and inserted into the operating channel with ease, targeting

Figure 2.15 Plastic cannulas can be used for intrauterine flushing (right) or instillation of high-viscosity fluid (left) (Cook Ob/Gyn)

Figure 2.16 Hysteroscopic corkscrew (7-Fr diameter) for myoma stabilization and removal (Cook Ob/Gyn)

the area without much manipulation of the hysteroscope itself. Alternatively, there are other forceps designed for operative hysteroscopy that can be used when sturdier instruments are required – the so-called optical forceps or optical scissors (Figure 2.14). These are assembled in the hysteroscope and cannot be moved unless the whole hysteroscope is moved. While these rigid instruments perform better when cutting or grasping or during biopsy, care should be taken to control their action at all times under panoramic view and to introduce them only under direct vision. The panoramic view of the uterine cavity may be impaired as they are fixed to the end of the endoscope and cannot be moved independently. These rigid optical instruments should be used selectively and only in special situations (Figures 2.15 and 2.16).

While most operative procedures with a hysteroscope are performed with flexible or semirigid instrumentation, electroprobes can also be used to coagulate or divide tissues. Differently shaped electroprobes are available (Figure 2.17), and their use requires the same precautions as when using electricity in any other part of the body.

New instrumentation has been designed to simulate the bipolar system by the construction of electrodes that deliver and recover the electrical current at a short distance, producing vapor pockets that control the energy and vaporize tissue in the pathway and, therefore, do not maintain as much erraticity of the energy, should the uterus be distended with fluids containing electrolytes. When employing monopolar electrosurgery, only fluids devoid of electrolytes can be used to avoid erratic dispersion of the electricity and perhaps even damage to other organs, as the current has to be increased to obtain some type of superficial tissue damage. However, the new systems of vaporization that permit the use of electrolytes certainly decrease the threshold for toxicity of fluids and avoid acute hyponatremia altogether. Additionally, should the fluid absorbed by the patient be excessive, more than a liter and a half, then diuretics can be used liberally to avoid fluid overload without triggering hyponatremia. These devices can be used through an operative hysteroscope or a small-caliber hysteroscope with an operating channel. The electrodes are designed in different shapes such as twizzle-type or thin

Figure 2.17 Ancillary electrode tips for hysteroscopy are available in various configurations (left to right): needle, ball, loop and hook (Cook Ob/Gyn)

wire, or ball shaped, depending on the tissue to be treated.

LIGHT SOURCES

Most light sources are the halogen type of 300–400 W. When video systems are used, it is important to have a light source that can provide adequate illumination to obtain the best resolution. Ideally, xenon or a halide light source should be used. Nonetheless, with the new high-sensitivity light cameras (three-chip cameras), the need for powerful light sources has markedly decreased. It is important, however, to replace the fiberoptic cables transmitting the light when breakage of fibers is observed by illuminating a surface directly with a light-transmitting cable.

BASIC INSTRUMENTATION IN HYSTEROSCOPY

Not many instruments are required for hysteroscopy, but it is important to have the correct instruments available during an examination.

For diagnostic hysteroscopy, a telescope and a diagnostic sheath with a diameter < 4 mm are necessary, as well as plastic tubing to conduct the CO_2 gas, a fiberoptic light-transmitting cable, a vaginal speculum to visualize the cervix, soft sponges for disinfection, a tonsil needle with an appropriate syringe to perform a paracervical block and a long tenaculum to stabilize the cervix.

Operative hysteroscopy requires a telescope 4 mm in outer diameter, a hysteroscopic bridge with a sheath 7–8 mm in outer diameter, plastic nipples to occlude the inner and outer ports, semirigid instrumentation including scissors, biopsy forceps and grasping forceps, and soft polyethylene catheters with an inner diameter of 1.67 mm and an outer diameter of 2.42 mm to permit selective cleansing of the uterine cavity. A video-camera recorder is most useful during diagnostic hysteroscopy, and is necessary during operative hysteroscopy not only for documentation, but also because it permits easier and more comfortable operation for the endoscopist. In addition, it provides excellent magnification and resolution of various tissues, enhancing the ease and precision of the procedure, and allows the assisting team to observe and assist with the operation.

CLEANSING AND MAINTENANCE OF INSTRUMENTS

After use, the endoscopes, hysteroscopes and resectoscopes and their components should be thoroughly rinsed and washed with special brushes and soaps. The ports and channels should be delicately cleaned with soft wire brushes and rinsed appropriately.

Disinfection and sterilization

While most instruments can be disinfected with solutions such as glutaraldehyde (Cidex®), overnight gas sterilization is the most commonly used method to sterilize safely and maintain the instruments ready for use. However, this solution over time may damage the optics and the cement gluing their parts. An autoclave can be used for all metallic parts except the telescope, plastic nipples and flexible plastic-coated instruments. The flexible hysteroscope needs cleaning, disinfection and sterilization with gas only. During storage, it is important to avoid dropping, bumping or bending these delicate instruments. The telescope should be kept in a separate container to avoid breakage.

One of the innovations in sterilization of these endoscopic instruments has been the introduction of a low-temperature sterile processing system such as the STERIS 1® with continuous, microcomputer-controlled monitoring of the sterilization procedure. Peroxyacetic acid (PAA) or peracetic acid is employed in a wide variety of antimicrobial applications in health care and in the food and beverage industry, combined with sterile water at pressure 40–50 psi (276–345 kPa) and rate flow 4 gal/min (15 L/min) at a temperature of 110–118°F (43–48°C). Because the process is rapid, usually 30 min, this method not only prevents damage to the telescopes but also provides a practical method of sterilizing in a short period of time the instrumentation for reuse.

An alternative to this method of sterilization is use of the new autoclaveable telescopes that can be sterilized quickly in standard autoclave systems.

SELECTED BIBLIOGRAPHY

Baggish MS. A new laser hysteroscope for Nd–YAG endometrial ablation. *Laser Surg Med* 1988;8:248

Brueschke EE, Wilbanks GD. A steerable fiber-optic hysteroscope. *Obstet Gynecol* 1974;44:273

Garner FM. Optical physics with emphasis on endoscopes. In Baggish MS, ed. *Gynecologic Endoscopy and Instrumentation*, Vol. 26. *Clinical Obstetrics and Gynecology*. Hagerstown, MD: Harper & Row, 1983: 213–18

Hamou J. Microhysteroscopy. A new procedure and its original applications in gynecology. *J Reprod Med* 1981;26:375

Hopkins HH. Optical principles of the endoscope. In Berti G, ed. *Endoscopy*. New York: Appleton-Century-Crofts, 1976:3–26

Iglesias JJ, Sporer A, Gellman AC, Seebode JJ. New Iglesias resectoscope with continuous irrigation, simultaneous suction, and low intravesicle pressure. *J Urol* 1975;114:929

Lin BL, Miyamoto N, Tomatsu M, et al. Flexible hysterofiberscope. The development of a new flexible hysterofiberscope and its clinical applications. *Acta Obstet Gynaecol Jpn* 1987;39:649

McCarthy JF. A new type observation and operating cystourethroscope. *J Urol* 1923; 10:519

Parent B, Guedj H, Barbot J, Nodarian P. *Panoramic Hysteroscopy* [English translation]. Baltimore, MD: Williams & Wilkins, 1987

Prescott R. Optical principles of endoscopy. *J Med Primatol* 1976;5:133

Quint RH. The rigid hysteroscope. In Sciarra JJ, Butler JC, Speidel JJ, eds. *Hysteroscopic Sterilization*. New York: Intercontinental Medical Book Corporation, 1974:11–18

Valle RF, Sciarra JJ. Current status of hysteroscopy in gynecologic practice. *Fertil Steril* 1979;32:619

Valle RF. Hysteroscopy for gynecologic diagnosis. In Baggish MS, ed. *Gynecologic Endoscopy and Instrumentation*, Vol. 26. *Clinical Obstetrics and Gynecology*. Hagerstown, MD: Harper & Row, 1983:253–76

Valle RF. Future growth and development of hysteroscopy. In DeCherney AH, ed. *Hysteroscopy, Obstetrics and Gynecology Clinics of North America*. Philadelphia, PA: WB Saunders, 1988:111–26

Valle RF. Office hysteroscopy. *Clin Obstet Gynecol* 1999;42:276-289

3

Uterine distention: media and techniques

For panoramic hysteroscopy, the uterine walls that are normally in apposition must be separated to create a true cavity (Table 3.1). The urinary bladder can easily be distended with gravity pressure. The thin distensible walls and epithelial lining do not change cyclically. As it is lined with a simple cuboidal epithelium, the bladder is an ideal organ for distention during cystoscopy. Furthermore, the urinary bladder has a much greater capacity than the uterus, and there is no communication between the bladder and the peritoneal cavity. For these reasons, cystoscopy can easily be performed without special equipment to distend the bladder.

In contrast, the uterus has thick muscular walls that require positive pressure for its distention. The uterine lining comprises cylindrical columnar epithelium that changes during each monthly cycle; the thickness, consistency, structure and vascularization make the performance of hysteroscopy particularly cumbersome in the luteal phase. The uterine cavity communicates directly with the peritoneal cavity, should fluid enter the Fallopian tubes. It is important, therefore, to understand the possible sequelae and pay attention to details when converting this potential cavity into an actual one. This is why hysteroscopy took longer than cystoscopy to become established as a practical technique.

MEDIA FOR UTERINE DISTENTION

Three different types of media can be used safely and effectively to distend the uterus:

Table 3.1 Factors related to panoramic endoscopy of the uterus and urinary bladder

Uterus	Urinary bladder
Virtual cavity with thick muscle walls	Thin muscle walls are easily distensible
Positive pressure needed for distention	Distensible with only gravity pressure
Bleeds at monthly cycles	No cyclical bleeding
Has columnar epithelium with glands	Has transitional epithelium
Epithelium changes cyclically	No cyclical changes
Communicates with peritoneal cavity via	No communication with
Fallopian tubes	peritoneal cavity
Has individual embryology, anatomy,	Has different embryology, anatomy,
physiology and pathology	physiology and pathology

CO_2 gas; low-viscosity fluids; and high-viscosity fluids.

CO_2 gas

The use of CO_2 gas requires electronic monitoring of the intrauterine gas pressure and the rate at which the gas is delivered (Figure 3.1). CO_2 gas is highly diffusible and soluble, permitting the continuous elimination of small quantities of intravasated gas by the lungs, using the enormous buffer capacity of the blood circulation as gas is continuously intravasated. With excessive amounts of intravasation, particularly if excessively high flow rates are used and if the intrauterine pressure markedly exceeds the mean arterial pressure, decompensation may occur. Therefore, it is important to use machines specifically designed for hysteroscopy which can calibrate not only the flow of the gas to around 40–50 ml/min, but also intrauterine pressure (not to exceed 150 mmHg). Most hysteroscopic examinations can be performed at a flow rate of approximately 30–40 ml/min with intrauterine pressure at approximately 60–70 mmHg. These two parameters compensate each other to maintain a proper balance. When the intrauterine pressure increases, the flow rate decreases, and vice versa.

CO_2 gas insufflation has several advantages. It is a 'clean' medium, permitting excellent visualization as there is no interposition of a substance to cause refraction, and adequately maintains distention of the uterine cavity. Nonetheless, there are some disadvantages, particularly when used for operative procedures. If CO_2 gas is mixed with blood, it may produce bubbling, which is cumbersome and may obscure the view. Because CO_2 gas is invisible, a leak in the system may not be noticed for some time. A spe-

Figure 3.1 An electronic hysterosufflator for uterine distention with CO_2 gas (upper); and an electronic pump for uterine distention with low-viscosity fluid (lower) (Storz)

cific machine is required for electronic calibration of the CO_2 flow rate and pressure. Finally, use of a laser becomes cumbersome owing to the smoke and fumes that cannot be easily evacuated without deflating the uterine cavity. However, it remains a good choice for diagnostic hysteroscopy as it uses small hysteroscopes < 4 mm in outer diameter that do not require cervical dilatation.

Low-viscosity fluids

Low-viscosity fluids are useful during operative procedures as they permit not only

Figure 3.2 (Left) Automatic pump for optimal fluid control (Olympus). (Right) Automated fluid monitoring pump (ACMI)

washing of the uterine cavity, but also lavage of the blood clots and debris that may form during an operation. These fluids are of two types: those containing electrolytes; and those that do not. Low-viscosity fluids containing electrolytes, specifically sodium in the form of sodium chloride (NaCl), are used when operative procedures are performed with mechanical tools or lasers that require no electricity. The presence of electrolytes makes the procedure somewhat safer and prevents hyponatremia, should excessive amounts of fluid be used and absorbed. The quantity of fluid used should be carefully monitored, with measurement of the amount of fluid instilled and recovered to permit estimation of the amount of fluid absorbed by the patient (Figure 3.2).

The most commonly used electrolyte-containing fluids for uterine distention are normal saline (0.9% NaCl), dextrose 5% in 50% saline solution (0.45% NaCl) and Ringer's lactate solution. All are equally effective in distending the uterine cavity and providing good visualization. Because these fluids are usually packaged in plastic bags containing 1000 ml, some positive pressure is necessary to distend the uterus adequate-

ly as gravity pressure is not sufficient under these circumstances. Alternatively, a mechanical pump such as those that measure fluid pressure and flow rate can be used, limiting the intrauterine pressure to no more than 100–120 mmHg. Nonetheless, even with such pumps, special care should be taken to monitor inflow and outflow to estimate the amount of unrecovered fluid.

While the use of isotonic fluids with electrolytes is permitted, with the systems mimicking a bipolar system, it is important to remember that excessive saline solution, if not monitored, may still produce pulmonary edema. Furthermore, when excessive saline solutions are used and the urine output is not well monitored, the patient may excrete hypertonic saline and instigate what is known as a desalination process. This process involves the excretion of hypertonic urine, usually accompanied by sodium and potassium, and liberation of free water in the intravascular tree that not only may contribute to pulmonary edema but also may produce a delayed hyponatremia. Therefore, it is important to monitor and determine precisely the amount of fluid not recovered, and if this is excessive, say,

1.5–2 L, evaluation of electrolytes must be carried out and instruction given to the patient upon discharge to report any unusual symptom or sequela such as disorientation or persistent nausea or vomiting, as these sequelae may be delayed 18–24 h after the procedure.

Low-viscosity fluids without electrolytes are required during electrosurgery with either the hysteroscope or resectoscope. Electrolytes are excellent conductors, but may disperse the electrical output erratically so that the desired effect on tissues may not be safely obtained. These fluids include dextrose 5% in water, glycine 1.5%, sorbitol 3%, a combination of sorbitol 2.8% and mannitol 0.5% and, finally, a mannitol 5% solution. Despite some differences in the osmolality of these substances, for practical purposes and for visualization, there are no major differences. Ideally, the solution should not change either plasma osmolality or plasma electrolytes; because these fluids contain no electrolytes, hyponatremia may occur if excessive amounts are absorbed by the patient. Mannitol 5%, an osmotic diuretic, decreases this risk; nonetheless, in the acute state, sodium may be lost and, therefore, careful monitoring of these patients is required.

Most of these substances, particularly glycine and sorbitol, are packaged in 3 liter plastic containers. If large-bore or urological tubing is used, and the bags are elevated above the patient to approximately 80 cm, then enough pressure is obtained to deliver these fluids by gravity alone, permitting adequate distention of the uterine cavity without the need for tourniquets or pumps. To obtain this effect, which is feasible with all resectoscopes, only hysteroscopes with continuous-flow systems are appropriate.

Low-viscosity fluids offer several advantages. They can clear debris, mucus and blood clots from the operative field and continuously wash the uterine cavity, permitting good visualization. Should the mechanism be faulty and leakage of fluid occur, it will be immediately visible, and the fluid instilled and recovered can easily be measured. Because these fluids, particularly those without electrolytes, may be intravasated, care should be taken to monitor meticulously the amount of fluid not recovered to alert the practitioner to intravasation and absorption by the patient. Although low-viscosity fluids may cross the Fallopian tubes, in general, the amount needed to distend the uterus is small and should not cause serious problems in the patient. In addition, when fluids without electrolytes are used, fluid deficits should be carefully monitored, as well as serum sodium, in view of the possibility of hyponatremia when excessive absorption occurs.

Ancillary equipment to monitor recovery of low-viscosity fluids

Plastic pouches can be modified and added to drapes or attached to the patient to permit adequate collection of fluid (Figure 3.3). These pouches are attached to special suction machines via large-port tubes that permit accurate recovery of this fluid into calibrated containers to measure the total outflow (Figure 3.4).

High-viscosity fluids

The most commonly used high-viscosity fluid is dextran with a high molecular weight (MW) – 70 000 MW – in a 10% water solution. This medium is highly viscous and, therefore, only small amounts are usually

Figure 3.3 Pouch for collecting fluid

Figure 3.4 Fluid management system with an electronic pump for use in an office or operating suite

required for an examination as the flow is slow on entering or exiting the uterine cavity. Dextran provides excellent visualization due to its high refractory index, and offers an excellent alternative to distention of the uterus when bleeding occurs in the uterine cavity, as it does not mix with blood.

Usually, examination can be performed despite a small amount of bleeding. Because dextran is a hyperosmotic solution, intravasation of excessive amounts may precipitate serious effects, such as pulmonary edema of non-cardiogenic origin and even coagulopathies due to changes produced in the cascade of coagulation factors. Dextran, however, is not used frequently at present.

Although it is evident that some type of mechanical pump is necessary to deliver these fluids safely and effectively, as yet, there is no such pump that is practical, totally safe and inexpensive. Specific intrauterine transducers are necessary for adequate measurement of intrauterine pressure, flow rate and the amounts of fluid injected, recovered and potentially absorbed by the patient.

TECHNIQUES FOR UTERINE DISTENTION

Panoramic hysteroscopy

For diagnostic or operative hysteroscopy, the patient is placed on an appropriate table in a dorsal lithotomy position. A bimanual pelvic examination is performed

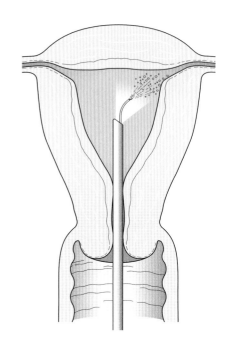

Figure 3.5 Position of a diagnostic endoscope (upper; 4 mm in outer diameter) compared with an operative hysteroscope (lower; > 6 mm in outer diameter) for examination

Figure 3.6 Flushing the uterine cavity using a polyethylene catheter inserted through the operative channel of a hysteroscope

to assess uterine size and direction. After proper disinfection of the vagina and vulva, a vaginal speculum is put into position and a paracervical block performed, if necessary. The anterior lip of the cervix is grasped with a single-tooth tenaculum. When using a diagnostic hysteroscope, the endoscope attached to its light source and the CO_2 gas distending medium is introduced at the level of the ectocervix before performing the systematic examination (Figure 3.5).

CO_2 gas hysteroscopy

When using CO_2 gas, it is important to check and calibrate the hysterosufflator

machine that delivers the CO_2 gas or liquid to ensure that there is an adequate reserve of gas and that the machine is working properly. A plastic tube is attached to the hysteroscope and, with the stopcock open, the flow rate is monitored. Gas pressure is recorded by the machine on opening and closing of the stopcock.

Hysteroscopy with low-viscosity fluids

With low-viscosity fluids, only hysteroscopes that permit continuous flow should be used. Before distention of the uterus, the uterine cavity should be cleared of debris, blood clots and mucus by a continuous-flow system or by inserting a

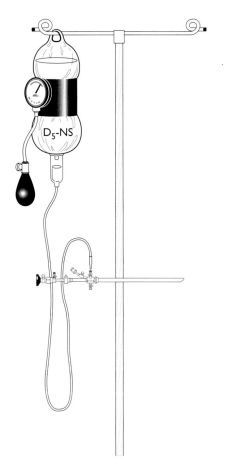

Figure 3.7 Instillation of fluids into the uterus using a plastic bag with a pressure cuff

the polyethylene catheter is clear, uterine distention can begin (Figure 3.7).

Hysteroscopy with high-viscosity fluids

When using high-viscosity fluids such as dextran, it is important to reload the 50-ml syringes with the fluid and to prime the tubes by injecting the fluid until it appears at the end of the syringe. Once the tube is attached to the hysteroscope, an assistant may slowly press on the plunger of the syringe until the uterus distends. The hysteroscopist may ask the assistant to increase the pressure as necessary, depending on the examination and visualization. It is important with high-viscosity fluids to wash the instruments immediately after their use to prevent caramelization or hardening of the dextran around the instrument as this may 'freeze' the stopcocks and locks of the instruments, making them inoperable. This method is seldom used at present.

PRACTICAL CONSIDERATIONS FOR TECHNIQUE AND EXAMINATION

Most scopes have a foreoblique view (25–30°; Figure 3.8). The standard position of the hysteroscope is with the light cord facing downwards so that the direction of view is upwards; thus, the anterior wall of the cervix is seen more clearly than the posterior wall (Figure 3.9a), and the opposite when a retroverted uterus is encountered (Figure 3.9b). The resectoscope has the light cord facing upwards so that the direction of view is somewhat downwards to observe the fitted electroprobe.

To introduce the scope, a slow side-to-side motion can be used and, once the

polyethylene catheter through the operative channel (Figure 3.6). Such cleansing is important, because most procedures performed with low-viscosity fluids are operative procedures using hysteroscopes which are 7–8 mm in outer diameter and almost always require cervical dilatation. If smaller diagnostic hysteroscopes with continuous-flow systems are used, then the continuous-flow system of the hysteroscope may be sufficient to cleanse the uterine cavity. Once the uterine cavity has been cleansed and the fluid retrieved through

Figure 3.8 The direction and angle of view changes with the shape (angle) of the distal lens

Figure 3.9 Visualization of the uterine cavity with a foreoblique lens: with the light cord facing downwards (a), the anterior wall is better visualized; when the light cord faces upwards (b), the posterior wall is better seen

uterine cavity is reached, this rotational motion can be increased in a clockwise or counterclockwise direction to observe the cornual regions and tubal openings. This rotational motion is not necessary with flexible endoscopes which compensate for the foreoblique view by allowing the tip of the instrument to be steered or bent towards the area under observation. Flexible hysteroscopes are introduced with the distal tip pointing straight ahead and are bent only while in the uterine cavity, or when entering a markedly anteflexed or retroflexed uterus. If a myoma or adhe-

sion interferes with the panoramic view of the uterine cavity or with the initial introduction, these instruments can be driven in by bending the distal tip to accommodate the endoscope to the particular distortion.

SELECTED BIBLIOGRAPHY

Baggish MS. Distending media for panoramic hysteroscopy. In Baggish MS, Barbot J, Valle RF, eds. *Diagnostic and Operative Hysteroscopy. A Text and Atlas.* Chicago, London, Boca Raton: Year Book Medical Publishers, 1989:89–93

Edstrom K, Fernstrom I. The diagnostic possibilities of a modified hysteroscopic technique. *Acta Obstet Gynecol Scand* 1970;45:327

Lavy G, Diamond MP, Shapiro B, DeCherney AH. A new device to facilitate intrauterine instillation of dextran 70 for hysteroscopy. *Obstet Gynecol* 1987;70:955

Lindemann HJ. The use of CO_2 in the uterine cavity for hysteroscopy. *Int J Fertil* 1972;17:221

Neuwirth RS, Levine RV. Evaluation of a method of hysteroscopy with the use of 30% dextran. *Am J Obstet Gynecol* 1972;114:696

Porto R, Gaujoux J. Une nouvelle méthode d'hysteroscopie, instrumentation et technique. *J Gynecol Obstet Biol Reprod* 1972;1:691

Quinones-Guerrero R, Alvarado-Duran A, Aznar-Ramos R. Histeroscopia. Una nueva tecnica. *Ginecol Obstet Mex* 1972;32:337

Quinones RG. Hysteroscopy: choosing distending media. Int J Fertil 1984;29:129

Shirk GJ, Kaigh J. The use of low-viscosity fluids for hysteroscopy. *J Am Assoc Gynecol Laparosc* 1994;2:11

Valle RF, Sciarra JJ. Present status of hysteroscopy in gynecologic practice. *Fertil Steril* 1979;32:619

Valle RF. Hysteroscopy for gynecologic diagnosis. *Clin Obstet Gynecol* 1983;26:253

Valle RF. Hysteroscopy. In Wynn RH, ed. *Obstetrics and Gynecology Annual*. New York: Appleton-Century-Crofts, 1978:245–83

4

Indications and contraindications of hysteroscopy

Before performing any surgical procedure, there must be a specific indication and the benefits obtained by the operation should greatly outweigh the potential risks. The appropriate technique and instrumentation should be established and defined, and there should be no contraindications to the procedure.

The potential applications of hysteroscopy were realized at its inception about a century ago, and its true value has been established by clinical trials which have confirmed the benefits and utility of hysteroscopy in clinical practice. At present, the main indication of its use is to evaluate abnormal uterine bleeding. Furthermore, pathological lesions such as polyps, submucous leiomyomas or focal areas of endometrium suggestive of hyperplasia or carcinoma can be identified, and their location, extension and particular topography assessed to allow determination of the need for selected biopsies or direct treatment (Table 4.1).

ABNORMAL UTERINE BLEEDING

Abnormal uterine bleeding is the main indication for hysteroscopy, particularly in premenopausal women with persistent abnormal bleeding, and bleeding in peri- and postmenopausal patients (Table 4.2). Direct visualization of the uterine cavity increases the accuracy of diagnoses of suspected intrauterine pathology by offering the opportunity to obtain selected biopsies of abnormal or suspicious areas of endometrium. Although suction aspiration of the endometrium is used routinely in the evaluation of patients with abnormal uterine bleeding, the accuracy and completeness of this evaluation may be limited in the presence of submucous leiomyomas or endometrial polyps and focal areas of endometrium, particularly at the uterotubal junctions. Direct visualization of the uterine cavity enhances evaluation of topographical and architectural distortions, allowing visual exploration of the entire uterine cavity.

Table 4.1 Diagnostic applications of hysteroscopy

Exploration of endocervical canal
Suspected endometrial polyps
Suspected submucous leiomyomas
Misplaced foreign bodies
Uterine anomalies
Intrauterine adhesions
Evaluation of endometrial lining
Evaluation of uterotubal junctions
Focal pathologically suspect lesions (endometrial carcinoma and precursors), location, extent

Table 4.2   Indications for hysteroscopy

Evaluate unexplained abnormal uterine bleeding in pre- or postmenopausal patients
Diagnose and/or transcervically remove submucous leiomyomas or polyps
Locate and retrieve 'lost' intrauterine devices and other foreign bodies
Evaluate infertile patients who have abnormal hysterosalpingograms
Diagnose and/or surgically treat intrauterine adhesions
Diagnose and/or surgically treat uterine septa
Explore endocervical canal and uterine cavity in cases of repeated spontaneous abortions
Evaluate failed first-trimester elective abortion
Ablate endometrium in intractable menorrhagia
Cannulate Fallopian tubes
Perform tubal sterilization

Hysteroscopy permits targeted biopsies to be taken of abnormal or suspicious areas of endometrium. Because visualization alone cannot adequately distinguish between benign and malignant or premalignant endometrial lesions, biopsies of these lesions are particularly important. In young adolescent patients complaining of abnormal uterine bleeding, the diagnosis can easily be obtained with a clinical history and selected laboratory evaluations to rule out coagulopathies; in adults and particularly those who are peri- or postmenopausal, however, endometrial biopsies are mandatory.

Although investigation of patients with abnormal uterine bleeding must be individualized, some fundamentals apply generally. A history and physical examination may suffice in adolescents; however, even in these patients, a pregnancy test using a rapid sensitive serum assay should be done to rule out pregnancy.

Essential laboratory tests should include a complete blood count, peripheral blood smear and a coagulation profile (bleeding time, platelet count, prothrombin time, partial thromboplastin time) to rule out coagulopathies. Serum progesterone, luteinizing hormone, follicle stimulating hormone, prolactin and thyroid stimulating hormone levels should be obtained to rule out most of the endocrinopathies that cause abnormal uterine bleeding. If hyperandrogenism or chronic annovulation is suspected, testosterone, dehydroepiandrosterone sulfate and 17-hydroxyprogesterone determinations are in order. Finally, structural disorders of the uterus such as submucous leiomyomas, polyps and endometrial abnormalities, including endometrial carcinoma and its precursors, must be ruled out. Intrauterine evaluation with hysteroscopy and appropriate biopsies is required. While the latter evaluation may not be required in adolescents unless they fail to respond to appropriate hormonal therapy, it becomes mandatory in adult women, particularly perimenopausal patients, to rule out any organic etiology of the abnormal bleeding. Because postmenopausal women, particularly those who present with uterine bleeding, are at greater risk of carcinoma than younger women, uterine evaluation is of the utmost importance. To facilitate a quick and appropriate uterine evaluation in postmenopausal women, an endometrial biopsy performed by suction in the office setting is appropriate. Should the biopsy detect pathology, appropriate therapeutic

Table 4.3 Hysteroscopic confirmation of hysterographic abnormal findings

Author	Patients with abnormal hysterograms (n)	Confirmed by hysteroscopy (%)
Edstrom and Fernstrom	30	53.3
Englund et al.	21	50.0
Gribb	14	43.0
Levine and Neuwirth	11	50.0
Norment	50	60.0
Porto and Serment	76	58.0
Sugimoto and Nishimura	206	65.0
Taylor and Cumming	68[*]	55.5
Valle	63	68.3
Varangot et al.[†]	71	55.0

[*]Normal hysterograms, only 30 confirmed
[†]Contact hysteroscopy

(From Valle and Sciarra, 1979)

measures should then be established. When the biopsy is negative for pathology, an ultrasound with or without fluid enhancement, depending on the findings, may be the second stage, to rule out endometrial polyps, myomas or focal thickened endometrium. If the ultrasound is negative with an endometrial stripe of less than 4 mm, hormonal manipulation will usually resolve the problem. Nonetheless, if there is no response, hysteroscopy should be added to rule out any missed lesion. If the ultrasound scan shows positive lesions in the uterine cavity, then hysteroscopy should be added to confirm and assess the proper diagnosis, with target biopsies, if required. The postmenopausal woman with abnormal uterine bleeding, therefore, requires complete and meticulous evaluation of the uterus and adnexa to rule out anatomical conditions such as polyps, myomas, adenomyosis, abnormal endometrium and associated adnexal pathology of the tubes and ovaries that may harbor pathology responsible for abnormal bleeding (Table 4.3, Figure 4.1).

Figure 4.1 Algorithm for evaluation of postmenopausal uterine bleeding

Table 4.4   Comparison of hysteroscopy and hysterosalpingography

Hysteroscopy	Hysterosalpingography
Direct visualization of uterine cavity	Indirect visualization (uses contrast-medium shadow)
Diagnosis and specification of intrauterine lesions	Recognition and presumptive diagnosis of intrauterine lesions
Possibility of targeted biopsy and surgical therapy	No possibility of targeted biopsy and surgical therapy
Precise localization of abnormalities (polyps, leiomyomas, malformations, adhesions, carcinomas and precursors)	Localization of abnormalities is less precise
Direct access to tubal lumen (biochemical or biophysical studies, selective chromopertubation)	No direct access (indirect study; possible spasm)
No evaluation of Fallopian tubes possible	Evaluation of tubal lumen, patency, epithelial folds and abnormalities
Requires special instrumentation and experience, and is more costly	Simple instrumentation, easy to perform and less expensive

INFERTILITY

Although hysteroscopy is not used routinely to evaluate infertility, it is the best method for confirming or rectifying an abnormal hysterosalpingogram. The latter method of evaluation has a significant rate of false-positives due to transient distortion of the uterine cavity owing to blood, mucus, debris and/or air bubbles. Confirmation of an abnormal hysterosalpingogram by subsequent hysteroscopy has varied from 43 to 68% in comparative studies (Table 4.3).

The abnormal hysterogram is the main indication for hysteroscopy in infertile patients. Hysteroscopy and hysterosalpingography do not exclude each other, but rather are complementary (Table 4.4). The hysterosalpingogram is the basic screening method for evaluating the uterine cavity and Fallopian tubes in the infertile patient. The method is relatively simple and inex-

pensive, and provides valuable information. When an abnormal hysterosalpingogram is obtained, it is important not only to confirm, but also to determine accurately, the abnormality and plan for treatment. Although, occasionally, hysteroscopy may detect minor abnormalities in a patient with a normal hysterogram, these findings are usually of minor or no clinical significance except when the endometrium is evaluated in patients with abnormal uterine bleeding.

Similarly, an abnormal sonogram dictates intrauterine visualization to confirm and/or treat any intrauterine lesion suspected by sonography.

SUSPECTED ENDOMETRIAL POLYPS AND SUBMUCOUS LEIOMYOMAS

Hysteroscopy is the best method for diagnosing or confirming endometrial polyps or

Figure 4.2 Hysteroscopic view of an endometrial polyp

Figure 4.3 Submucous leiomyoma with characteristic peripheral vascularization seen through an atrophic endometrium

submucous leiomyomas. Endometrial polyps are due to proliferation and hypertrophy of the basal layer of the endometrium. On visualization, the polyp surface shows virtually no vascularization (Figure 4.2) as most vascularization is central, branching peripherally from a central core. The polyps are smooth and soft, and indent easily on contact. Submucous leiomyomas are benign solid tumors composed of muscular fibers and fibrotic connective tissue; in general, except when they have a necrotic surface, they show a peculiar superficial vascularization that is visible through atrophied endometrium (Figure 4.3) which can easily be traced to the base of the myoma. When these superficial vessels are injured, they bleed profusely as they lack a muscular wall hemostatic mechanism. They feel hard to the touch and cannot be indented easily with probes and forceps. Both types of lesions may be sessile or pedunculated (Figure 4.4) and located at different levels of the uterine cavity. Because these lesions

Figure 4.4 This sessile submucous leiomyoma was located in the left lower portion of the uterine cavity

distort the symmetry of the uterine cavity, they are easily diagnosed on panoramic visualization of the uterine cavity with a hysteroscope.

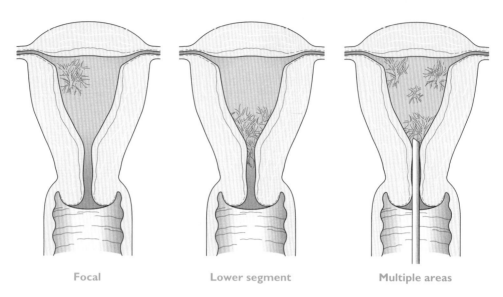

Focal   Lower segment   Multiple areas

Figure 4.5   Various presentations of intrauterine adhesions

SUSPECTED INTRAUTERINE ADHESIONS

Scars resulting from trauma in the postpartum or postabortal period may cause menstrual abnormalities such as hypomenorrhea and amenorrhea, depending on the extent of uterine cavity occlusion. The diagnosis is usually suspected from the patient's history and confirmed by hysterosalpingography. To outline the precise distortion of the uterine cavity and permit direct treatment, intrauterine visualization is required. With hysteroscopy, the uterine cavity can be evaluated and its symmetry re-established with selective division of the adhesions.

To determine the prognosis in the treatment of intrauterine adhesions, it is important to classify the extent of uterine cavity occlusion (Figure 4.5) and the types of adhesions present. Using hysterosalpingography and hysteroscopy, three types of intrauterine adhesions may be defined:

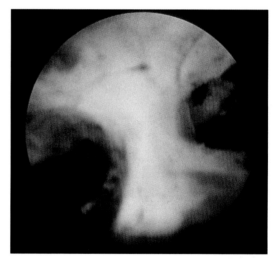

Figure 4.6   This thick adhesion extends from one uterine wall to the other, thereby causing distortion of the uterine cavity

mild adhesions are filmy (endometrial) adhesions which produce partial or complete uterine cavity occlusion; moderate adhesions are fibromuscular adhesions that are characteristically thick and covered

Figure 4.7 Thick connective-tissue adhesions occupying a large portion of the uterine cavity. Small area (3 o'clock) free of adhesions

Figure 4.8 Uterotubal cone with left tubal opening

with endometrium that may bleed upon division, and can partially or totally occlude the uterine cavity (Figure 4.6); severe adhesions are composed of connective tissue only with no endometrial lining, are unlikely to bleed upon division and may partially or totally occlude the uterine cavity. The more fibrotic are the adhesions, the worse is the prognosis and, thus, the thinner and more recent are the adhesions, the better is the prognosis (Figure 4.7).

EVALUATION AND CONFIRMATION OF UTERINE ANOMALIES

Uterine septa

Approximately 25% of women with a septate uterus experience reproductive wastage. The classical clinical picture is that of repeated early mid-trimester abortions with signs of labor and bleeding. By tradition, when women with repetitive abor-

tions due to uterine septation require treatment, abdominal metroplasty either by excision of the septum through a wedge uterine excision (Jones) or by incision of the septum without excision of tissue (Tompkins) has been performed. Both operations require laparotomy and hysterotomy, with their concomitant inconvenience, hospitalization and prolonged recovery.

Uterine septa may vary in length, be either partial or complete, or involve the cervix as well. Septal thickness varies from thin to thick and wide. Furthermore, when uterine septa are present, other uterine pathology, such as polyps, myomas or intrauterine adhesions, may be encountered.

Because uterine septa are often poorly vascularized, hysteroscopy is used to divide the septum transcervically under direct vision; the procedure was previously attempted blind by a few practitioners, but abandoned owing to the difficulties involved.

31

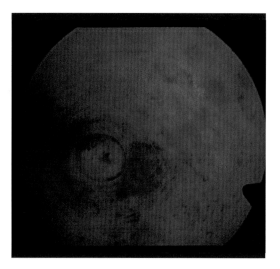

Figure 4.9 Right uterine horn with tubal opening

Figure 4.10 Hysteroscopic view of the uterotubal junction

Tubal ostia

The first 2–3 mm into the tubal ostia can be evaluated by hysteroscopy. Although partial tubal cannulation was first performed in the late 1960s, the technique was not refined until the early 1970s, with experience gained from tubal sterilization. Hysteroscopic evaluation of the intramural Fallopian tubes provides an opportunity to treat polyps and adhesions obstructing or distorting the tubal ostia. Because the first 2–3 mm of the Fallopian tube is not markedly convoluted, direct ostial cannulation, performed since the early 1970s, allows the selective assessment of tubal patency (Figures 4.8 and 4.9).

Several pathological conditions may be diagnosed at the tubal openings. These include polyps occluding the tubes, adhesions, and rigid or sclerotic tubal ostia that do not respond well to stimuli and produce physiological spasms that may inhibit opening and closing with intrauterine pressure. The first 2–3 mm of tubal epithelium can also be visualized and evaluated by hysteroscopy (Figures 4.10–4.12).

OTHER CLINICAL APPLICATIONS

Hysteroscopy is of value in exploring the cervical canal in patients who have had repeated abortions. Visual appraisal of the cervical canal during hysteroscopic examination reveals that, in many of these patients, there is a loss of the anatomical relationship between the corpus and the cervix, and disappearance of the sphincter-like action of the internal cervical os. Uterine anomalies can also be detected. Of late, hysteroscopic tubal sterilization has become a reality, with ESSURE microinserts placed at the intramural portion of the Fallopian tubes and proximal isthmic tubal segments.

Adenomyosis

Adenomyosis is difficult to diagnose consistently with hysteroscopy and is only occasionally suspected if small sinuses are observed, particularly in the fundal region. The condition is also difficult to diagnose by

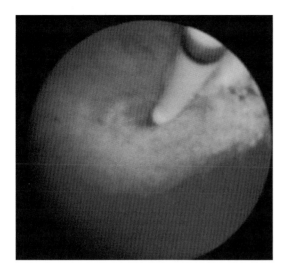

Figure 4.11 Hysteroscopic cannulation of the tubal ostium

Figure 4.12 Chromopertubation shows tubal patency at laparoscopy after cannulation

biopsy taken through the hysteroscope or even with the resectoscope, as only superficial myometrial tissue can thus be obtained. The best method available for the diagnosis of adenomyosis is magnetic resonance imaging (MRI), particularly if the patient reports abnormal uterine bleeding and cyclical pain, although vaginal ultrasound can measure myometrial thickness.

Tubaloscopy

Tubaloscopy has been attempted since the late 1960s, using the hysteroscope as the conduit for miniendoscopes or fallopo-scopes; manufacturers are now developing new miniendoscopes that improve the field of view and resolution, and also offer the capability of washing and introducing fluids while maintaining a diameter of less than 1 mm. The miniendoscope is still being investigated and cannot be routinely used for transcervical evaluation of the Fallopian tubes.

Although the ability to examine the tubal lumen from the uterine side has developed with the introduction of hys-teroscopy, achieving a clear and distinct view of the tubal lumen has been difficult due to the limitations of technology. It is possible to pass small catheters into the tubal lumen, but the view obtained with microendoscopes is poor, with low resolution. Such small-diameter endoscopes cannot provide adequate flushing and disten-tion of the tube to permit the endoscope to be advanced from the uterus.

The best evaluation is obtained during withdrawal of the endoscope. Endoscopy of the ampulla and distal end of the tube is best performed with rigid endoscopes 3 mm in diameter introduced from the abdominal side. This permits excellent distention and visualization, thereby allowing the recogni-tion and evaluation of these anatomical structures.

Tubal endoscopy from the uterus remains a research tool waiting for technol-ogy to provide the appropriate endoscopes to allow clear and distinct evaluation of the structures and topography of the intramural and isthmic tubal lumen.

Embryoscopy

Although it is possible to introduce miniendoscopes transcervically to observe the early embryo, the optical resolution has not been satisfactory. Rigid miniendoscopes can now be introduced transabdominally and transuterinally to observe the embryo *in situ* with better resolution. As the technology advances, the possibility of a practical transcervical method for embryoscopy remains on the horizon. As miniendoscopes become accepted for intrauterine visualization, the transfer of gametes, zygotes or embryos under visual control may become a reality.

The fundamental elements needed to perform hysteroscopy on the embryo include an appropriate hysteroscope, a uterine-distending medium, an illumination source and ancillary instrumentation.

When an early first-trimester pregnancy termination fails and histological examination of the products of conception does not demonstrate chorionic villi, an ectopic pregnancy should be suspected, particularly if the pregnancy test is persistently positive. When laparoscopy fails to demonstrate tubal pathology and/or lesions of the ovary or peritoneal layer consistent with an ectopic pregnancy, hysteroscopy may be of value. The reason may be early gestation in an anomalous uterus, such as a septate uterus with an early pregnancy at a site that was not curetted. Hysteroscopy can guide selective suction aspiration for termination of the missed pregnancy. This approach has been greatly facilitated with the use of concomitant sonography.

Although the indications of hysteroscopy are well established, other potential hysteroscopic diagnostic applications remain under investigation. Changes in topography of the endometrium during the menstrual cycle have been evaluated by correlation of superficial vascularization patterns and changes in the endometrial glandular openings as the cycle progresses with the degree of endometrial maturation. Miniaturization of endoscopes permits less traumatic access for tubal cannulation of the Fallopian tubes, and may open the door to better evaluation of the Fallopian tubes and to applications for new reproductive technologies. Tubal sterilization using microinserts is now a reality and applied in the clinical setting.

In summary, the most common indications for hysteroscopy are: evaluation of abnormal, persistent or recurrent uterine bleeding; evaluation of an abnormal hysterogram; surgical treatment of intrauterine adhesions; division of uterine septa; removal of submucous leiomyomas; location and removal of misplaced intrauterine devices; tubal cannulation in patients with tubal cornual occlusions; and endometrial ablation (destruction).

CONTRAINDICATIONS OF HYSTEROSCOPY

Some contraindications are absolute in that hysteroscopy should never be performed when these contraindications are present. Others are relative, and indicate that the technique must be modified and patients individually selected for this approach.

Absolute contraindications are pelvic inflammatory disease and profuse uterine bleeding. Pelvic inflammatory disease is an absolute contraindication because of the potential of spreading infection, through either the bloodstream or lymphatic routes systemically, or Fallopian tubes into the peritoneal cavity. Infection must be ruled out in patients presenting with symptoms or a history of recent pelvic infection by appropriate cervical cultures before hysteroscopy to prevent exacerbation of an existing infection, and by applying meticulous attention to technique to avoid introduction of new infection to the endometrial cavity.

Profuse uterine bleeding can make hysteroscopy cumbersome regardless of the distending medium used. If bleeding is not excessive, proper evacuation and washing of the endometrial cavity prior to uterine distention may permit adequate, albeit temporary, visualization.

Relative contraindications are desired pregnancy, cervical malignancy, menstruation, known adenocarcinoma of the endometrium, cervical stenosis, recent uterine perforation and operator inexperience.

Pregnancy

Hysteroscopy is contraindicated during pregnancy, as the possibility of infection or interruption of a wanted pregnancy far outweighs the value of intrauterine observation. Nonetheless, under special circumstances, such as removal of misplaced intrauterine devices in early pregnancy, visualization may be performed in selected patients, with the technique modified to decrease the chances of interrupting the pregnancy. It is important to weigh the benefits derived from hysteroscopy during early pregnancy against the potential of damaging or interrupting the pregnancy.

Cervical malignancy

In the presence of known cervical malignancy, manipulation of the area should be avoided to prevent possible spread. Patients with known carcinoma of the cervix should not be subjected to hysteroscopy particularly because the information derived may not contribute to the plan of treatment. Nonetheless, under meticulous and controlled protocols, the endocervical canal can be evaluated with a small-caliber endoscope to assess the extent of an adenocarcinoma of the cervix. This evaluation should be carried out in conjunction with a gynecological oncologist to establish a proper plan of therapy.

Menstruation

Hysteroscopy should not be performed during menstruation to avoid potential risks of infection from necrotic tissue; menstrual blood could potentially be pushed through the Fallopian tubes into the peritoneal cavity by distention. However, if necessary, hysteroscopy could be performed with a continuous-flow hysteroscope that permits continuous washing of blood and debris under low intrauterine pressures to avoid transtubal reflux. Hysteroscopy is best performed following the completion of menstruation.

Adenocarcinoma of endometrium

Hysteroscopy is used in the evaluation of patients with abnormal uterine bleeding. Occasionally, abnormal focal areas of endometrium are found and confirmed to be carcinomas. However, in a patient with known carcinoma of the endometrium, the use of hysteroscopy should be cautiously undertaken particularly because, at that stage, a carcinoma is likely to be extensive, and adding hysteroscopy may not change the plan of treatment. If it is necessary to determine involvement of the cervix, hysteroscopy may be used in collaboration with a gynecological oncologist to evaluate the extent of the adenocarcinoma and confirm involvement of the cervical canal. However, following the new FIGO (International Federation of Gynecologist and Obstetricians) Guidelines for surgical staging, this evaluation has become unnecessary.

Cervical stenosis

When the endocervical canal cannot be dilated adequately to introduce the endoscope, hysteroscopy cannot be performed. With the use of small-caliber endoscopes, the procedure may be facilitated, but if the endoscope, despite a small caliber, cannot be passed through the cervical canal under direct vision, the procedure cannot be performed safely.

Recent uterine perforation

If the uterus cannot be distended adequately due to a uterine wall defect, hysteroscopy becomes cumbersome. The patient should be allowed to heal and the examination performed at a later time. Nonetheless, perforation with a small-caliber endoscope may not preclude uterine distention if appropriate precautions are taken. When a small perforation has occurred, hysteroscopy may be attempted with a continuous-flow system to permit continuous lavage. If this does not permit uterine distention, then laparoscopy may help in occluding the small perforation from the abdominal side while hysteroscopy is being performed. However, previous healing of the defect will permit better evaluation of the uterine cavity.

Operator inexperience

Attempting hysteroscopy without proper training and supervision may convert a simple technique into a potential source of complications. Of all the contraindications, that of greatest concern is cervical or uterine infection without obvious clinical symptoms. Fortunately, active infection following hysteroscopic examination is rare. Nonetheless, strict adherence to a combination of proper indications, absence of contraindications, meticulous technique and an experienced surgeon pave the way for a procedure performed without serious complications or sequelae.

SELECTED BIBLIOGRAPHY

Ahumada JC, Gandolfo-Herrera R. Histeroscopia. *Rev Med Lat Am* 1935;21:265

Bordt J, Belkien L, Vancaillie T, *et al*. Ergebnisse diagnostischer hysteroskopien in einem IVF/ET-Programm. *Gerburts Frauenheilkd* 1984;44:813

Ghilardini G, Gualerzi C, Fachi F, *et al*. Chorionoscopy and chorionic villi sampling. *Acta Eur Fertil* 1986;17:491

van Herendael B, Stevens M, Flakiewicz-Kula A, Hansch C. Dating of the endometrium by microhysteroscopy. *Gynecol Obstet Invest* 1987;24:11

Kerin J, Dayhovsky L, Segalowitz J, *et al*. Falloposcopy: a microendoscopic technique for visual exploration of the human fallopian tube from the uterotubal ostium to the fimbria using a transvaginal approach. *Fertil Steril* 1990;54:390

Lin J, Chen YO, Lin BL, Valle RF. Outcome of removal of intrauterine devices with flexible hysteroscopy in early pregnancy. *J Gynecol Surg* 1993;9:195–200

Mencaglia L, Ricci G, Perino A, *et al*. Hysteroscopic chorionic villi sampling: a new approach. *Acta Eur Fertil* 1986;17:495

Menken FC. Endoscopic observations of endocrine processes and hormonal changes. In Ruiz-Albretch F, Ramirez-Sanchez J, Willowitzer H, eds. *Simposio sobre Esteroides Sexuales*. Berlin: Saladruck, 1969:276

Norment WB. Hysteroscope in diagnosis of pathological conditions of uterine canal. *J Am Med Assoc* 1952;148:917

Norment WB, Sikes CH, Berry FX, Bird I. Hysteroscopy. *Surg Clin North Am* 1957;37:1377

Novy MJ, Thurmond AS, Patton P, *et al*. Diagnosis of cornual obstructions by transcervical fallopian tube cannulation. *Fertil Steril* 1988;50:434

Pantaleoni DC. An endoscopic examination of the cavity of the womb. *Med Press Circ* (Lond) 1969;8:26

Quinones-Guerrero R, Alvarado-Duran A, Aznar-Ramos R. Tubal catheterization: applications of a new technique. *Am J Obstet Gynecol* 1972;114:674

Quinones-Guerrero R, Aznar-Ramos R, Alvarado-Duran A. Tubal electrocauterization under hysteroscopic control. *Contraception* 1973;7:195

Sciarra JJ, Butler JC, Speidel JJ, eds. *Hysteroscopic Sterilization*. New York: Intercontinental Medical Book Corporation, 1974

Sciarra JJ, Valle RF. Hysteroscopy. A clinical experience with 320 patients. *Am J Obstet Gynecol* 1977;127:340

Snowden EU, Jarret JC, Dawood MY. Comparison of diagnostic accuracy of laparoscopy, hysteroscopy, and hysterosalpingography in evaluation of female infertility. *Fertil Steril* 1984;41:709

Valle RF, Sciarra JJ. Current status of hysteroscopy in gynecologic practice. *Fertil Steril* 1979;32:619

Valle RF. Hysteroscopic evaluation of patients with abnormal uterine bleeding. *Surg Gynecol Obstet* 1981;153:521

Valle RF. Hysteroscopy in the evaluation of female infertility. *Am J Obstet Gynecol* 1980; 137:425

Valle RF, Sabbagha RS. Management of first trimester pregnancy termination failures. *Obstet Gynecol* 1989;73:201

Valle RF. Future growth and development of hysteroscopy. In DeCherney AH, ed. *Hysteroscopy*. Philadelphia, PA: WB Saunders, 1988: 111–26

Valle RF. Indications for hysteroscopy. In Siegler AM, Lindemann HJ, eds. *Hysteroscopy: Principles and Practice*. Philadelphia, PA: JB Lippincott, 1984:21–4

Valle RF. Hysteroscopy for gynecologic diagnosis. In Baggish MS, ed. *Gynecologic Endoscopy and Instrumentation. Clinical Obstetrics and Gynecology*. Hagerstown, MD: Harper & Row, 1983:253–76

Valle RF. Hysteroscopic sterilization with the ESSURE system. In Sciarra JJ, ed. *Gynecology and Obstetrics. Fertility Regulation, Psychosomatic problems, Infertility, Genetics*, Vol. 6, Ch. 40. New York: Lippincott-Raven 2004:1–40

5

Possible complications of hysteroscopy

Because hysteroscopy is a surgical technique requiring manipulation of the cervix and uterus, and dissection and removal of intrauterine pathological lesions, it has the potential for complications. These complications may be related to the procedure itself, distending medium, specific surgical procedures performed, additional techniques or instrumentation that may be required or to the anesthesia.

PROCEDURAL COMPLICATIONS

Complications related to the procedure itself are similar to those that occur during intrauterine manipulations such as curettage. These include laceration of the cervix by a tenaculum, uterine perforation and infection. Cervical laceration from the tenaculum can occur when excessive manipulation is performed by traction, but can easily be corrected by suturing the defect and prevented by gentle manipulation. While minor lacerations can occur while placing the tenaculum in the cervix, bleeding can occur only if the uterine walls are damaged or a vascular tumor is disturbed. Uterine perforation can occur either during blind uterine sounding or cervical dilatation before hysteroscopy or when the hysteroscope is advanced blindly and forcibly into the uterine cavity. This type of perforation can be prevented by not advancing the endoscope unless a panoramic view is accomplished by adequate uterine distention. The use of a uterine sound is seldom required as the endoscope is guided under direct vision. Cervical dilators should not be advanced beyond the internal os.

When these complications occur, the treatment varies according to the size and location of the perforation. Perforation with a uterine sound seldom requires treatment (Figures 5.1–5.3). If a uterine perforation occurs, the procedures of hysteroscopy should be avoided altogether and the patient observed for possible decompensation. When uterine perforation is due to a large operative hysteroscope, further evaluation may be necessary, including laparoscopy to assess persistent bleeding and to accomplish hemostasis. During operative procedures, should perforation occur with mechanical instrumentation, the treatment usually does not differ from perforations due to the hysteroscope itself. If perforation occurs when additional techniques such as electrosurgery or a laser are used, further evaluation is mandatory to rule out damage to adjacent structures. If laparoscopic evaluation is negative, patients should be followed closely for signs of infection, early intestinal obstruction and/or delayed hemorrhage.

Figure 5.1 Posterior uterine perforation by a uterine sound

Figure 5.2 Anterior uterine perforation by a uterine sound in a retroverted uterus

Infection, although possible when an endoscope is introduced into the uterine cavity, is rare when precautions such as disinfection and sterilization of instruments are taken. The appropriate selection, evaluation and preparation of patients for hysteroscopy helps to prevent infection. To avoid contamination of the cervical canal and uterine cavity during the procedure, sterile techniques should be maintained and protocols meticulously followed.

COMPLICATIONS WITH DISTENDING MEDIA

Complications related to distending media vary according to the medium. When CO_2 gas exceeds the flow rate of 100 ml/min, hypercapnia, arrhythmias, acidosis and even gas emboli may occur. These problems can be avoided by using machines specifically designed for hysteroscopy which electronically calibrate the appropriate flow rate of about 40–60 ml/min and do not permit

Figure 5.3 Fundal perforation by a uterine sound

intrauterine pressures > 100–150 mmHg. Other machines not specifically designed for hysteroscopy, particularly those used for laparoscopy, should never be used to distend the uterus. When low-viscosity fluids are used to distend the uterine cavity during operative hysteroscopy, the most frequent complications are secondary to fluid overload and electrolyte imbalance, particularly if fluids devoid of electrolytes are used. It is important, therefore, to control meticulously the quantity of fluids administered and to measure the quantity of fluids recovered. Furthermore, the intrauterine pressure should be kept below the mean arterial pressure of 100 mmHg (Figure 5.4).

Although there is no specific standard quantity of non-recovered fluids or deficit that is absolutely safe, several parameters alert the endoscopist to early decompensation. When fluids with electrolytes are used, the threshold of toxicity or decompensation may be increased, as significant diuresis may compensate for the fluid overload in the early stages. When prolonged procedures are performed and significant dissections are required, it is important to measure urine output with an indwelling catheter to assure no oliguria or anuria occurs. The anesthesiologist should carefully monitor vital signs such as blood pressure, pulse and pulse oximetry. The circulating nurse should meticulously measure the fluid introduced or injected as well as the fluid recovered to have an accurate periodic account of the deficit.

Fluids containing electrolytes are less likely to cause serious problems. Fluid overload cannot be totally avoided, but precautionary measures such as early diuretic use can be implemented to prevent intravasation of excessive amounts of fluid. Hyponatremia is avoided and the threshold for toxicity increased as the patient maintains diuresis. In general, a deficit of no more than 1000–1500 ml of fluid containing electrolytes should be permitted. This amount, although conservative, will certainly prevent major fluid overload. If the quantity of non-recovered fluid detected is

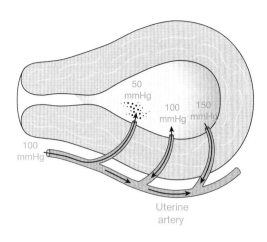

Figure 5.4 Titration of intrauterine pressure against mean arterial pressure

excessive, particularly with signs of decompensation in the vital signs, pulse oximetry or urine output, the operation should be stopped and diuretics administered under close monitoring.

When fluids devoid of electrolytes are used, precautions in addition to monitoring should be undertaken. Should a deficit of 800 ml occur, the operation should be stopped and a stat serum sodium determined. If no lowering of the serum sodium has occurred, the operation may proceed providing that only a short time is required to complete the procedure. However, if the serum sodium is lower than normal and the required operation is prolonged, the procedure should be aborted and completed at another time. Further decompensation in the serum sodium with deficits > 1000 ml should be immediately and appropriately corrected. The use of diuretics under these circumstances should be undertaken with caution and meticulous monitoring of serum electrolytes and urine output.

The outlined precautions of keeping a strict account of fluid deficits, particularly when devoid of electrolytes, during hysteroscopic and resectoscopic procedures, and ensuring attention to and surveillance of the patient's condition during these procedures by the anesthesiologist with pulse oximetry, vital signs, body temperature as measured by esophageal probes, cardiac rhythm and testing of electrolytes, particularly sodium as required, provide the basic evaluation of the patient necessary to diagnose early the possibility of fluid overload and its sequelae. When using fluids without electrolytes, however, early detection of hyponatremia cannot be completely guaranteed by measuring fluid deficits and other monitoring signs, as these may present late and therefore fail to signal initiation of fluid overload. Based on electronic chip computer monitoring technology, point-of-care testing of electrolytes can be accomplished in a short period of time, less than 2 min, utilizing only one or two drops of whole blood in the microchip chambers. This technology, now available worldwide, has been difficult to establish in most hospitals owing to fear of decentralization however, it is used in most emergency units and in cardiovascular surgery where immediate results are important. Several systems, used such as the I-STAT and others.

In order to make clinical decisions during hysteroscopic surgery regarding fluid absorption and early development of hypernatremia, immediate and frequent monitoring of electrolytes, particularly sodium, is of utmost importance. New technologies such as the I-STAT – a new standard in blood analysis – has made it possible for immediate, continuous, rapid monitoring of electrolytes in the operating room. By combining silicon chip manufac-

turing technology with classical electrochemistry, quick blood analysis without sacrificing accuracy and reliability is possible. The procedure provides immediate results that do not interrupt surgery, requiring a waiting time of less than 2 min. This new technology allows the surgeon to make critical decisions when performing resectoscopy procedures.

When using dextran 70 32% for operative procedures, it is important to measure the amount of dextran infused and the amount recovered to prevent more than 300 ml being absorbed by the patient. When greater quantities are absorbed by intravasation of the dextran under pressure, a non-cardiogenic pulmonary edema may occur, perhaps due to the osmotic effect of the dextran shifting fluids to the intravascular space. Additionally, because of the effect of dextran on coagulation factors, a coagulopathy similar to disseminated intravascular coagulation may ensue, with decreasing platelets, a prolonged partial thromboplastin time and low fibrinogen. This condition should be recognized and immediately treated with respiratory support measures, cautious use of diuretics and plasmapheresis for degradation of the large molecules of dextran; if coagulopathy ensues, appropriate therapy should be given. Allergic reactions to dextran, although unusual, may occur and require appropriate management. In such cases, the operation should be immediately discontinued, and the patient provided with therapeutic support of circulatory and respiratory systems.

If a procedure is expected to be prolonged, monitoring is mandatory. If the procedure cannot be completed with a limited amount of dextran, other alternatives should be instituted, including low-viscosity fluids with or without electrolytes, depending on the procedure and the type of energy used.

Embolism

CO_2 gas embolization may occur when the gas is used to distend the uterine cavity in an uncontrolled manner. New insufflation machines designed specifically for hysteroscopy electronically control the intrauterine pressure at no more than 150 mmHg and the rate of infusion at no more than 100 ml/min. The use of these units has practically eliminated the occurrence of CO_2 embolization. CO_2 laparoscopy insufflation machines should never be used for hysteroscopy, because they permit flow rates that are far too high for this procedure. If CO_2 embolism is suspected, immediate resuscitative measures are necessary. The patient should be placed on her left side, oxygen should be administered and direct percutaneous cardiac aspiration of gas should be performed. Room air embolism, although rare, can also occur through open uterine venous channels and sinuses. Thus, excessive use of the Trendelenburg position should be avoided, and hysteroscopy or resectoscopic cannulas should not be left open in the uterus while obturators, electrodes or telescopes are removed. Treatment measures for room air embolism are similar to those for CO_2 embolization. Should stabilization of the patient be achieved, hyperbaric oxygenation may be the most effective therapy for this condition.

COMPLICATIONS OF ANESTHESIA

Complications may be related to the anesthetic used. Local anesthetics may on occasion cause allergic reactions, but the most common complications are due to intravasation. Therefore, the type of anesthetic used, whether an ester or amide, should be known. The toxicity of these anesthetics should be kept in mind and, when problems of intravasation occur, they should be appropriately handled. Usually, intravenous diazepam corrects the problem. Anesthetics of the ester type, such as chloroprocaine (Nesacaine®) and mercaine, have a low toxicity and, when intravasation occurs, their rapid degradation by plasma pseudocholinesterase helps in their elimination. Because only a small amount is generally required for paracervical block, 3–4 ml in each uterosacral ligament, toxicity is markedly decreased.

Problems related to general anesthesia and regional anesthetics are the responsibility of the anesthesiologist.

COMPLICATIONS OF LASERS IN OPERATIVE HYSTEROSCOPY

When using fiberoptic lasers, it is important to use either the bare fiber, or sculpted or extruded fibers, and to avoid coaxial fibers, particularly those fitted with sapphire tips as they require continuous cooling by gases or fluids. Indeed, the latter lasers should never be used in the uterus to avoid massive intravasation of gas or air developing into a fatal gas embolus. When using these fine fiberoptic lasers to operate in the uterus, perforation of the uterine wall can occur if the laser is pressed too quickly into the uterine wall. Perforation can be avoided by operating at all times under direct view with great caution and attention to detail. If perforation occurs while the laser is activated, injury to other organs is possible. Because of the reflective nature of these lasers and their attraction to pigments, the operator and assistants should protect their eyes with special goggles or filters to avoid retinal injuries.

COMPLICATIONS OF ELECTROSURGERY

Electrosurgery may cause complications. Because a monopolar current is used, the patient should be properly grounded with an appropriate ground plate serving as a return electrode. Only insulated electrodes and probes should be used; the machines delivering this type of energy should be properly calibrated and have a display of the selected waveform and watt power. Electrosurgery should never be activated without a precise and complete view of the area to be treated, and only fluids devoid of electrolytes should be used to distend the uterine cavity.

COMPLICATIONS FROM OTHER PROCEDURES

Complications resulting from hysteroscopy vary according to the type of procedure performed. The most common complications related to hysteroscopic surgery are bleeding and uterine perforation. These can occur during division of uterine septa or intrauterine adhesions, treatment of myomas, endometrial ablation and tubal cannulation. Because some of these procedures require more time than others, it is important to monitor the fluids used during these procedures to prevent excessive absorption by the patient and fluid overload. Perforation of the uterus may also predispose the patient to injuries to other organs in the pelvic cavity. Therefore, when difficult procedures are performed, particularly if the symmetry of the uterine cavity is markedly distorted, concomitant laparoscopy or sonography are a helpful adjunct to prevent additional injuries to adjacent organs should perforation occur. While infection with this type of hysteroscopic procedure is uncommon, prophylactic antibiotics are selectively used in some patients, particularly those hoping to preserve fertility by treatment of septa, adhesions and tubal cannulation.

Ideally, no complications should follow any procedure or, when they occur, they should be justified by the need for and benefits derived from the procedure to respect the dictum of *primum non nocere*. Close attention to technique, selection of patients, avoidance of contraindications and appropriate performance of each procedure is of utmost importance.

SELECTED BIBLIOGRAPHY

Arieff AI, Ayres JC. Endometrial ablation complicated by fatal hyponatremic encephalopathy. *J Am Med Assoc* 1993;270:1230

Baggish MS, Brill AF, Rosenzweig B, *et al.* Fatal acute glycine and sorbitol toxicity during operative hysteroscopy. *J Gynecol Surg* 1993;9:137

Gallinat A. The effect of carbon dioxide during hysteroscopy. In van der Pas H, van Herendael BJ, van Lith DAF, Keith LG, eds. *Hysteroscopy.* Boston, The Hague, Dordrecht, Lancaster: MTP Press, 1983:19–27

Garry R, Hasham F, Kokri MS, Mooney P. The effect of pressure on fluid absorption during endometrial ablation. *J Gynecol Surg* 1992;8:1

Hulka JF, Peterson HB, Phillips JM, Surrey MW. Operative hysteroscopy. American Association of Gynecologic Laparoscopists 1991 membership survey. *J Reprod Med* 1993;38:572

Loffer FD. Complications from uterine distention during hysteroscopy. In Corfman RS, Diamond M, DeCherney A, eds. *Complications of Laparoscopy and Hysteroscopy*. Oxford, London, Edinburgh: Blackwell Scientific Publications, 1993:177–86

McLucas B. Hyskon complications in hysteroscopic surgery. *Obstet Gynecol Surv* 1991;46:196

Nachum Z, Kol S, Adir Y, Melomed Y. Massive air embolism – a possible cause of death after operative hysteroscopy using a 32% dextran 70 pump. *Fertil Steril* 1992;58:836

Peterson HB, Hulka JF, Phillips JM. American Association of Gynecologic Laparoscopists 1988 membership survey on operative hysteroscopy. *J Reprod Med* 1990;25:590

Valle RF. Cervical and uterine complications during insertion of the hysteroscope. In Corfman RS, Diamond M, DeCherney A, eds. *Complications of Laparoscopy and Hysteroscopy*. Oxford, London, Edinburgh: Blackwell Scientific Publications, 1993:167–76

Valle RF. Complications of hysteroscopy: prevention, recognition, and management. In Ransom SB, Dombrowski MP, Evans MJ, Ginsburg KA, eds. *Contemporary Therapy in Obstetrics and Gynecology*. Philadelphia, PA: WB Saunders, 2002:383–86

Witz CA, Silverberg KM, Burns WN, *et al.* Complications associated with the absorption of hysteroscopic fluid media. *Fertil Steril* 1993;60:745

6
Diagnostic and therapeutic hysteroscopy in the office

Office hysteroscopy became practical with the introduction of small-caliber endoscopes (< 4 mm outer diameter) permitting its use in the office setting without the need for cervical dilatation. The small-caliber hysteroscope simplifies examination and allows an easy, safe and expeditious investigation of the uterine cavity. Nonetheless, the small-caliber endoscope has inherent drawbacks. Initially, operative instruments could not be passed through these small hysteroscopes and only CO_2 gas could be used for uterine distention. However, these small hysteroscopes allowed diagnostic hysteroscopy to be performed quickly and simply without the need for anesthesia and/or analgesia.

Thus, the hysteroscope used in an office setting can only serve diagnostic purposes (Figure 6.1). The distending medium is CO_2 gas delivered by a hysterosufflator that electronically maintains the flow rate at a constant $40–50$ ml/min and permits an intrauterine pressure of no more than

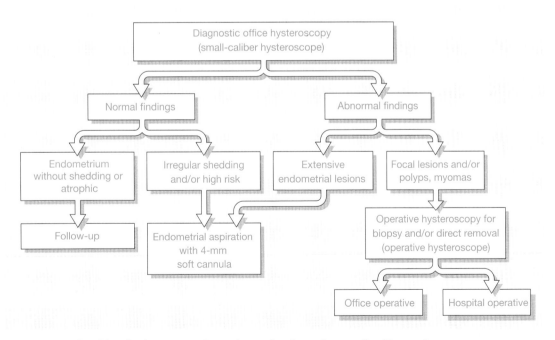

Figure 6.1   Algorithm for hysteroscopic uterine evaluation using small-caliber endoscopes

Figure 6.2 Fluid management system simplified for uterine distention in the office (ACMI)

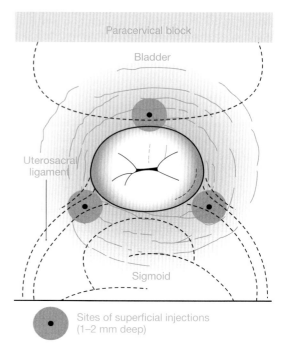

Figure 6.3 Sites of superficial injections (1–2 mm in depth) of anesthetic for a paracervical block

100–150 mmHg when the Fallopian tubes are open. As the intrauterine pressure increases, the flow rate decreases, and vice versa. While endoscopes with an outer diameter > 4 mm have been developed for use in the office, they are cumbersome; cervical dilatation is often necessary and the patient requires more local anesthetic or sedation. The cervical canal is traumatized, and the uterine cavity may contain debris and blood clots that cause the CO_2 gas to bubble inside the cavity, obscuring the view. Whereas endoscopes with diameters > 4 mm provide a system for washing the cavity with fluids, this method is also cumbersome in the office due to the additional tubing and collection bags for the fluid. Only if the system is simplified and adapted to individual settings can the latter method be an option for office hysteroscopy (Figure 6.2). Small-caliber hysteroscopes with 5-Fr operative channels permit minor therapeutic procedures in the office setting.

The patient selected for hysteroscopy requires a pelvic examination, and disinfection of the vagina and cervix with an antiseptic solution such as povidone iodine (Betadine®). In general, no systemic sedatives or medications are required as the procedure is practically painless. A paracer-

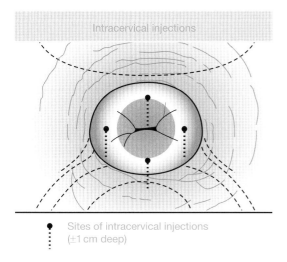

Figure 6.4 Intracervical injections are approximately 1 cm in depth

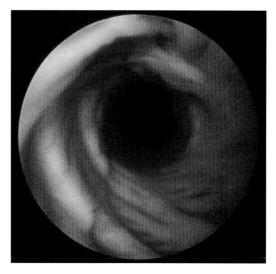

Figure 6.5 Hysteroscopic view of the cervical canal

vical block with 3–4 ml of a local anesthetic, preferably an ester type such as chloroprocaine hydrochloride (Nesacaine® 1%), is injected at the base of each uterosacral ligament, close to the cervix and superficially so as to blanch when injected to avoid rapid diffusion (Figure 6.3). A small amount (0.5 ml) at the site where the tenaculum is to be placed is useful (Figure 6.4). Once this is accomplished, a hysteroscope with its light source and flowing CO_2 gas or fluid is introduced under direct vision to the level of the ectocervix, and the examination begins by slowly and systematically following the small microcavity produced by the CO_2 gas or fluid in front of the endoscope. Once the endocervical canal is completely explored (Figures 6.5 and 6.6), the endoscope is advanced across the internal cervical os to allow evaluation of the panoramic view of the uterine cavity, including the uterotubal cornua and tubal ostia. The uterine cavity is re-examined, as is the endocervical canal, during withdrawal of the instrument.

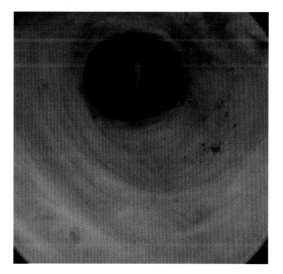

Figure 6.6 Closer view of the endocervical canal

Because most of these examinations are diagnostic, any pathology found will require either biopsy or hysteroscopic removal. Should therapeutic hysteroscopy be needed, a larger instrument may be required. The decision as to whether this can be performed safely in the office, or in an ambulatory surgical center or operating room suite under local, regional or general anesthesia, will depend on the lesion treated. Patients with normal findings at diagnostic hysteroscopy are spared any other manipulation or biopsy. On completion of the hysteroscopic examination in patients with abnormal uterine bleeding but normal hysteroscopic findings, who nonetheless have abnormal irregular shedding of the endometrial lining as is usually the case in patients with abnormal uterine bleeding, a 4-mm soft plastic cannula is introduced and suction curettage performed for histological evaluation. Because the patient has had a paracervical block, this suction aspiration is usually well tolerated.

Hysteroscopy has been facilitated as a simple office procedure with the use of small-caliber endoscopes. Because of its simplicity and ease of application, hysteroscopy is useful as a screening method for patients with abnormal uterine bleeding and/or questionable hysterograms, and for patients with suspected intrauterine pathology.

Although hysteroscopy can be performed in an office using an operative hysteroscope with a 7-mm outer diameter, the required cervical dilatation and manipulation usually involves additional assistance and attention to detail as well as safety measures in anticipation of such side-effects as bradycardia and/or hypotension. The procedure is similar to that described for office hysteroscopy except that the endocervical canal is gradually dilated to the diameter of a number 7 Hegar (or whichever specific operative hysteroscope is to be used). Despite the feasibility of introducing an operative hysteroscope under paracervical block anesthesia, the

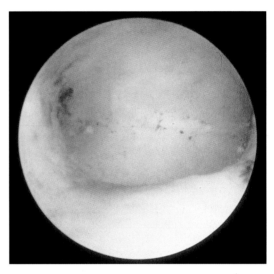

Figure 6.7 Hysteroscopic view of the uterine cavity in the early follicular phase

Table 6.1 Indications of operative hysteroscopy in office (vary according to experience and instrumentation)

Intrauterine devices and other foreign
  bodies removal
Endometrial biopsies
Small (< 2 cm) pedunculated polyps
Small (< 1 cm) pedunculated submucous
myomas
Lysis of focal and filmy intrauterine adhesions
Small (< 1 cm) uterine septa
Tubal sterilization (ESSURE™ microinserts)

operative procedures that can be safely performed in the office are limited to such procedures as removal of lost intrauterine devices (IUDs), biopsy of focal lesions, removal of small polyps and tubal occlusion procedures. The introduction of small-caliber hysteroscopes with 5-Fr operative channels has expanded these procedures (Table 6.1). Other manipulations and cervical interventions such as the division of extensive intrauterine adhesions or uterine

Figure 6.8 Hysteroscopic view of the uterine cavity in the secretory phase

Figure 6.9 Closer view of secretory endometrium. Observe cobble-stone appearance with deep glandular crypts

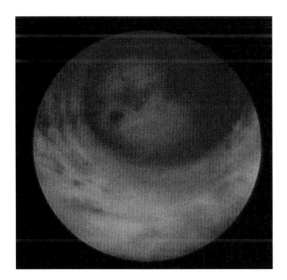

Figure 6.10 Hysteroscopic view of the uterine cavity in the postmenopausal woman shows atrophic endometrium

Figure 6.11 Atrophic endometrium (closer view)

septa, removal of submucous leiomyomas or endometrial ablation are more safely and effectively performed under regional or general anesthesia and, in some instances, with concomitant laparoscopy.

Office hysteroscopy is a simple procedure that can be undertaken in a short period of time with minimal morbidity and inconvenience to the patient. It is important to select the patient appropriately and

51

to schedule the examination during the follicular phase once menstruation is completed (Figures 6.7–6.11). In postmenopausal patients, the procedure can be performed when there is no bleeding. When plastic cannulas activated by suction are used for endometrial sampling, the combined procedures offer an excellent method for evaluation of patients with abnormal uterine bleeding, particularly when no focal pathology is found that requires selective, targeted biopsies. This method of evaluation is useful in premenopausal patients unresponsive to hormonal therapy and particularly peri- and postmenopausal patients with abnormal bleeding.

PRACTICAL POINTS FOR OFFICE HYSTEROSCOPY

Although the procedure of hysteroscopy is relatively simple, an important factor is to decrease patient anxiety and concerns by adequate instruction. Usually, a nurse or an assistant can describe hysteroscopy to the patient in lay terms and also help with the informed consent. Patients should be put at ease as much as possible by having the simplicity and rationality of the procedure explained. Furthermore, the use of a video system helps to explain findings. While a paracervical block is being performed, the patient should be kept informed as regards each step of the procedure. Ideally, an electrically driven examining table should be used to tilt or elevate the patient as required. A pelvic examination should be performed to determine the size of the uterus and its orientation. Once the speculum is placed to expose the cervix, the vagina and vulva are disinfected. Before any manipulation of the cervix is attempted, a paracervical block

should be performed and a tenaculum applied to the anterior lip of the cervix. The hysteroscope is introduced and the findings explained to the patient observing the video screen. Should a vabra-type aspiration biopsy be required, the procedure should also be explained to the patient. Occasionally, patients may require a non-steroidal anti-inflammatory agent following suction aspiration to relieve uterine cramps. The use of a vaginal speculum and tenaculum can be avoided in some patients by performing a vaginoscopic approach or insertion of the hysteroscope through a distended vagina with the fluid delivered by the hysteroscope.

Office procedures should be simple, expeditious and comfortable for the patient to achieve the full value of these procedures – decreasing expense and inconvenience to the patient and physician, and permitting better utilization of resources.

It is important, therefore, to have the appropriate instrumentation displayed and a special electrically driven table to move the patient into position without difficulty, with local anesthesia if required, a knowledgeable assistant, appropriate informed consent, and equipment for treatment of hypotension or other unwanted side-effects or problems requiring resuscitation measures.

CORRELATION OF DIAGNOSTIC HYSTEROSCOPY WITH HYSTEROSALPINGOGRAPHY, VAGINAL ULTRASOUND AND FLUID-ENHANCED SONOGRAPHY

Hysterosalpingography remains the initial screening method for evaluation of the uterine cavity and Fallopian tubes in infertile patients as it provides useful information regarding Fallopian tube anatomy and patency. The information derived from the hysterosalpingogram is particularly useful when normal findings are obtained. When the hysterosalpingogram reveals abnormalities, endoscopy becomes mandatory to confirm or rectify the abnormal picture. Indeed, around 30–40% of abnormal hysterographic findings may not be confirmed by direct visualization of the uterine cavity as the abnormalities may be due to debris, blood clots, mucus or transient distortion of the uterine cavity during performance of the procedure itself.

As only topography is evaluated by endoscopy, ultrasonography complements endoscopic evaluation by providing information about the uterine walls, indicating not only their thickness, but also the presence or absence of intramural or submucous leiomyomas. If central lesions are suspected of being polyps, or leiomyomas are encountered, additional evaluation may be obtained by injection of small quantities of fluid into the uterine cavity as contrast. This permits evaluation of any lesion that is intracavitary and reveals its extension into the uterine wall. Fluid-enhanced sonography does not permit either a panoramic view or anatomical evaluation of intrauterine lesions.

The blood flow of vascular structures such as myomas and polyps can be evaluated by Doppler ultrasonography to understand better their anatomy, physiology and malignant potential. This method, although promising, remains under evaluation. An abnormal sonogram, nonetheless, will require hysteroscopy for confirmation and/or treatment.

Magnetic resonance imaging (MRI) is useful in selected patients, particularly those harboring lesions not accurately evaluated by sonography, such as adenomyosis, and for uterine evaluation of obese women, particularly when vaginal/abdominal sonography is unsuccessful or inconclusive.

SELECTED BIBLIOGRAPHY

Barbot J, Parent B, Dubuisson JB. Contact hysteroscopy: another method of endoscopic examination of the uterine cavity. *Am J Obstet Gynecol* 1980;136:721

Bibbo M, Kleuskens L, Azizi F, *et al.* Accuracy of three sampling techniques for the diagnosis of endometrial cancer and hyperplasias. *J Reprod Med* 1982;27:622

Burnett JE. Hysteroscopy-controlled curettage for endometrial polyps. *Obstet Gynecol* 1964; 24:621

Englund SE, Ingelman-Sundberg A, Westin B. Hysteroscopy in diagnosis and treatment of uterine bleeding. *Gynecologia* 1957;143:217

Font-Sastre V, Carabias J, Bonilla-Musoles F, Pellicer A. Office hysteroscopy with small-calibre instruments. *Acta Eur Fertil* 1986;17:427

Goldchmit ZK, Blickstein I, Caspi B, Dgani R. The accuracy of endometrial Pipelle sampling with and without sonographic measurement of endometrial thickness. *Obstet Gynecol* 1993;82:727

Goldrath MH, Sherman AI. Office hysteroscopy and suction curettage: can we eliminate the hospital diagnostic D & C. *Am J Obstet Gynecol* 1985; 152:220

Gribb JJ. Hysteroscopy. An aid in gynecologic diagnosis. *Obstet Gynecol* 1960;15:593

Hamou J. Microhysteroscopy: a new procedure and its original applications in gynecology. *J Reprod Med* 1981;26:375

Karacz B. Office hysteroscopy. In Siegler AM, Lindemann HJ, eds. *Hysteroscopy: Principles and Practice*. Philadelphia, London, New York: JB Lippincott, 1984:106–7

Novak E. A suction-curette apparatus for endometrial biopsy. *J Am Med Assoc* 1935; 104:1497

Parent B, Guedj H, Barbot J, Nodarian P. In Meloine SA, ed. *Panoramic Hysteroscopy*. [English translation]. Baltimore, MD: Williams & Wilkins, 1985

Rodriguez GC, Yakub N, King ME. A comparison of the Pipelle device and Vabra aspiration as measured by endometrial denudation in hysterectomy specimens: the Pipelle device samples significantly less of the endometrial surface than the Vabra aspirator. *Am J Obstet Gynecol* 1993;168:55

Stock RJ, Kanbour A. Prehysterectomy curettage. *Obstet Gynecol* 1975;45:537

Valle RF. Hysteroscopic evaluation of patients with abnormal uterine bleeding. *Surg Gynecol Obstet* 1981;153:521

Valle RF. Hysteroscopy. In Garcia CR, Mastroianni L, Amelar RD, Dubin L, eds. *Current Therapy of Infertility*. Toronto, Philadelphia: BC Decker Inc., 1988:9–12

Valle RF. Future growth and development of hysteroscopy. In DeCherney AH, ed. *Hysteroscopy*. Philadelphia, London, Toronto, Montreal, Sydney, Tokyo: WB Saunders, 1988

Valle RF. Office hysteroscopy. *Clin Obstet Gynecol* 1999;42:276–89.

Word B, Gravlee LC, Wideman GL. The fallacy of simple uterine curettage. *Obstet Gynecol* 1958;12:642

7

Therapeutic hysteroscopy

Whether using local, regional or general anesthesia, the technique of operative or therapeutic hysteroscopy is similar to that of diagnostic hysteroscopy except that the endoscopes are larger, usually 7–8 mm in outer diameter, and, thus, usually require cervical dilatation. The uterine cavity is distended with low-viscosity fluids and, depending on the procedure, a medium with or without electrolytes is selected. When a tight and difficult-to-dilate cervical canal is encountered, an obturator attached to the outer sheath of the hysteroscope is used for the initial introduction, permitting insertion as far as the cervical os. The obturator is removed, and replaced by the scope and bridge. When low-viscosity fluids are used for uterine distention, a polyethylene catheter 2.4 mm in outer diameter and 1.6 mm in inner diameter may be introduced to the end of the hysteroscope before distention begins, should the continuous-flow system not cleanse the uterine cavity well (Figure 7.1). The fluid under pressure is allowed to enter the uterine cavity, permitting siphoning of the fluid through the polyethylene catheter.

When the distending medium exiting through the outflow port of the hysteroscope or the polyethylene catheter from the uterine cavity is clear of detritus, debris and blood clots, intrauterine visualization can begin. Targeted aspiration of selected areas of the uterine cavity may be performed with the polyethylene catheter to permit complete and unopposed visualization. If the operative hysteroscope has only one operating channel, the polyethylene catheter is removed to allow ancillary instruments to be inserted. Video cameras can be adapted for attachment to the ocular portion of the hysteroscope before insertion into the uterine cavity after adjustment for uniform color and a focused image. The correct orientation of the hysteroscope before insertion is with the fiberoptic light cable facing downwards, indicating that the viewing scope is facing upwards. The camera is kept in position without rotation; if rotation is required, only the hysteroscope should be rotated to observe the lateral aspects of the uterine cavity and tubal openings. When laparoscopy is used to monitor intrauterine surgery or for other reasons, the laparoscope is inserted first to allow uterine manipulation such as cervical dilatation or introduction of the hysteroscope aided by the laparoscopic view. To monitor hysteroscopic surgery, it is helpful to dim the light of the laparoscope to permit hysteroscopic illumination through the uterine wall. Innovations in instruments, light sources, video cameras, ancillary instrumentation and energy sources such as laser and electrosurgery have increased the therapeutic uses of hysteroscopy.

J.A.Ruiz/87

Figure 7.1 Flushing the uterus through a polyethylene catheter: (a) antero-posterior view, (b) lateral view

TARGETED BIOPSY

Among the therapeutic applications of hysteroscopy (Table 7.1) are targeted biopsies. Biopsies of the endometrium are initially obtained with suction devices, particularly of the Vabra type, to remove as much endometrial tissue as possible. This method has proved especially helpful in the evaluation of patients who have abnormal uterine bleeding and extensive areas of endometrium that need to be biopsied. However, when focal lesions of endometrium are present particularly at the uterotubal cornua and/or confined to polyps, or should submucous leiomyomas be present, these latter conditions may not be correctly diagnosed. Visual appraisal of the uterine cavity can provide accurate targeted biopsies of focal lesions that may be missed by the mechanical or suction devices available today. Specifically, endometrial polyps can easily be detected and extracted, and focal areas of endometrium biopsied directly, particularly those located at the uterotubal cornua where they can be easily missed by blind methods of evaluation. Endometrial lesions suspected of malignancy can be visually evaluated and a directed biopsy of an abnormal area performed. With the currently available hysteroscopic ancillary biopsy instruments, punch or spoon 5-Fr or 7-Fr forceps, only small portions can be obtained; it is therefore necessary to take

Table 7.1   Therapeutic applications of hysteroscopy

Targeted biopsy
Removal of endometrial polyps
Removal of submucous leiomyomas
Division of uterine septa
Removal of 'lost' intrauterine devices and other foreign bodies
Lysis of intrauterine adhesions
Endometrial ablation (laser, electrosurgery, hydrothermal)
Tubal cannulation (tubal obstruction, etc.)
Chorionic villus sampling
Tubal occlusion (electrocoagulation, cryocoagulation, chemical, mechanical, mechanical–ESSURE microinserts)

Figure 7.2   Pedunculated endometrial polyp

Figure 7.3   Dividing pedicle of polyp

several samples of the same area to have adequate tissue for histopathological evaluation.

REMOVAL OF ENDOMETRIAL POLYPS AND SUBMUCOUS LEIOMYOMAS

In the past, blind methods of evaluation and treatment were used when attempting the removal of polyps; forceps were introduced and opened blindly in the uterine cavity in an attempt to grasp a polyp. Such maneuvers were sometimes frustrating and inadequate. The visual appraisal of the uterine cavity provided by the hysteroscope offers an excellent method for the removal of polyps, particularly pedunculated polyps, which can be transected and removed in their totality (Figures 7.2–7.5). Sessile polyps can be also removed in this manner and the base treated by suction curettage. The resectoscope is particularly useful for removing this type of polyp as the

Figure 7.4 Endometrial polyp after removal

Figure 7.5 Large sessile polyp with resectoscopic loop behind for resection. Observe paucity and capillary-like aspect of superficial vessels

Figure 7.6 Hysterogram showing a uterine cavity deformed by a submucous tumor

Figure 7.7 Hysteroscopic view of a submucous leiomyoma

base can easily be resected in its totality to avoid recurrences. Whatever method is chosen for removal, it is important to ensure that the entire polyp has been removed, and this can only be confirmed visually by hysteroscopy. There are several alternatives for the removal of polyps, including blind attempts with a curette or polyp forceps once the polyp has been diagnosed and located.

Uterine leiomyomas are common neoplastic disorders that often require surgical treatment, particularly if they are submucous (Figures 7.6–7.10). Submucous myomas may invade the uterine wall virtually in their totality and show, like an iceberg, only a small tip of myoma in the cavity. This type

Figure 7.8 Hysteroscopic removal of a pedunculated submucous myoma using semirigid scissors

Figure 7.9 Myoma after removal

Figure 7.10 Hysterosalpingogram 3 months following myomectomy shows normal and symmetrical uterine cavity

Figure 7.11 Resection of a sessile submucous leiomyoma using a cutting loop

of myoma cannot be treated endoscopically and may even require a hysterotomy with uterine reconstruction, if symptomatic.

No blind method is useful in the treatment of submucous leiomyomas. Removal of these tumors must be accomplished via endoscopes, which require more experience to use. Several hysteroscopic methods are available to remove submucous leiomyomas (Figures 7.11–7.14). When a leiomyoma is

pedunculated and no greater than 3 cm in diameter, transection of the pedicle can be accomplished with mechanical hysteroscopic scissors; the cervix can be dilated and the myoma grasped with toothed forceps and removed transcervically. Most submucous leiomyomas are sessile and partly intramural, but most of the tumor is intraluminal. This type of tumor benefits most from resectoscopic shaving of the myoma, which causes the uterus to contract so that the myoma that is intramural becomes intraluminal, allowing its complete removal. However, this effect is noted only when the intraluminal

Figure 7.12 After complete resection of a myoma the fascicularis muscular layer at the right uterine wall is preserved

Figure 7.13 Hysterosonogram shows pedunculated submucous myoma

part of the leiomyoma is larger than the part that lies within the uterine wall. This can be assessed preoperatively by vaginal ultrasound complemented by fluid injection into the uterine cavity, so-called fluid-enhanced sonography. When the leiomyoma is sessile or has a broad pedicle, the best method of removal is by resectoscopy to shave systematically the leiomyoma from top to bottom until the myometrium is reached. (For more details on the technique of resectoscopic myomectomy, see Chapter 8.)

Visualization of the myoma surface will show peripheral vascularization through an atrophic endometrium as well as the whitish aspect of the fibrotic myoma tissue, as compared to the surrounding endometrium and myometrium. Tactile sensation with an inactivated loop will also provide a feel of the hardness of this tissue as compared to the soft fascicularis layer composed by the myometrium. The size of the radius of the cutting loop should be known, to enable application to the myoma surface according to the size of the intraluminal portion and to use shallow cuts when reaching the uterine surface. The loop upon activation

should elevate the tissue away from the uterine wall to avoid digging deeply into the myometrium.

While concomitant laparoscopy is not mandatory during myomectomy, the laparoscope should be used when resecting large submucous tumors that invade the myometrium deeply or when resection becomes difficult due to location, for example, at the uterotubal cornua.

With new advances in the use of the resectoscope, submucous myomectomy has been greatly facilitated and, at present, the gynecological resectoscope is the instrument of choice for these operations.

Results of hysteroscopic myomectomy

The resolution of abnormal bleeding in patients with submucous leiomyomas that do not harbor additional large intramural leiomyomas is impressive: over 95% of these patients obtain resolution of abnormal bleeding provided that the tumor is removed in its totality. Patients who have a portion of the leiomyoma left behind may require a second procedure to complete the myomectomy.

Figure 7.14 3-D fluid-enhanced sonography demonstrates an intramural myoma uterine cavity and endometrial polyp

Practical considerations in the treatment of myomas

Resection of endometrial polyps, particularly those of the sessile type, should be done systematically from the surface of the polyp to the uterine wall and with special attention paid to removing the totality of the basalis endometrium without shaving the myometrium, to prevent recurrences.

Uterine bleeding due to submucous leiomyomas may be evaluated by endometrial biopsy and ultrasound to determine the presence of other myomas as well as their number, size and location. In infertile patients, a hysterosalpingogram should be performed to determine the degree of distortion of the uterine cavity and condition of the Fallopian tubes, particularly when the leiomyoma arises from the cornual regions.

If the patient is anemic or there is continual marked bleeding, and if the leiomyoma markedly distorts the symmetry of the uterine cavity, it is useful to treat such patients with gonadotropin-releasing hormone (GnRH) analog to stop the bleeding, and decrease the vascularity of the tumor and its

volume. Three or more monthly injections of leuprolide acetate (depot Lupron®) 3.75 mg are required until the hemoglobin and hematocrit are normalized.

The leiomyoma is systematically shaved to the level of the uterine wall. The shavings of myoma are removed as they impair visibility, and the uterine cavity is re-examined to determine whether any protrusion of intramural leiomyoma still requires shaving. The tissue is visualized to identify the fascicularis layer of the myometrium from the fibrotic myoma tissue, and the cutting loop is activated to cut towards the operator while at all times elevating the leiomyoma from its bed. It is important to monitor the amount of fluid administered and recovered to calculate the deficit, and to attach an indwelling catheter to monitor urine output. If a difficult myomectomy is suspected, the patient should be prepared for laparoscopy.

UTERINE SEPTA

Uterine septa cause reproductive failure in about 25% of patients with this condition (Figure 7.15). These patients have repetitive pregnancy losses in the late first trimester or early second trimester with a minilabor, bleeding and abortion. When other reasons for the reproductive failure are excluded, these patients become good candidates for hysteroscopic surgery.

A thin uterine septum can be divided with hysteroscopic scissors whereas thick and broad septa require a sharp cutting electrode and the resectoscope (Figures 7.16–7.22). Division of these embryological remnants is performed under laparoscopic control to maintain uniform transillumination of the fundal portion of the uterus while the septum is being divided. Once the uterine cavity

Figure 7.15 Uterine septa range from partial to complete and may include vaginal septation (1–5)

Figure 7.16 Hysterosalpingogram showing a complete septum dividing the uterine cavity

Figure 7.17 3-D sonography shows a septate uterus

is symmetrical and both uterotubal cornua are visible, division is complete (Figures 7.23 and 7.24). Care must be taken to watch for bleeding after decreasing the intrauterine pressure by slowing the influx of distending medium. Selective coagulation is performed before the operation is concluded.

Three methods can be used to divide a uterine septum: hysteroscopic scissors; resectoscopic cutting electrodes; and fiberoptic lasers.

Treatment of uterine septum with hysteroscopic scissors

The uterine septum is usually divided hysteroscopically with semirigid scissors (Figures 7.25 and 7.26). The uterine septum, in general, is poorly vascularized; therefore, this technique is useful as division is along the midline, comprising the least vascular tissue and avoiding the anterior

Figure 7.18 Hysteroscopic view of a complete uterine septum

Figure 7.19 Complete uterine septum

Figure 7.20 Hysteroscopic septal division using semirigid scissors

Figure 7.21 Final sculpting of the fundal uterine wall using semirigid scissors

and posterior areas where bleeding can occur (Figures 7.27–7.29). The hysteroscopic division of a septum is performed with concomitant laparoscopy to monitor the amount of light shining through the translucent uterine wall. Division is performed systematically from side to side until the uterotubal openings can be seen and bleeding is observed at the myometrial junction. Once septal division is complete, the intrauterine

pressure of the distending fluid can be decreased; if arterial bleeding occurs, selective coagulation can be performed with a 7-Fr ball-tipped electrode. A medium without electrolytes such as glycine or sorbitol should be used. If bleeding has occurred, the resectoscope can be used to coagulate selectively each bleeding arteriole.

Figure 7.22 Hysterosalpingogram showing a symmetrical uterine cavity following treatment

Figure 7.23 Hysteroscopic view of a thick uterine septum

Figure 7.24 Division of the septum using a resectoscope

Figure 7.25 Completing the division of a broad septum with rectoscope

In general, the semirigid scissors perform efficiently, although if the septum is thick, then rigid scissors may be required. This latter instrument should be used with caution and under a perfect panoramic view particularly at the fundal area. Because flexible or semirigid hysteroscopic scissors are fragile and may not function properly at all times, a spare scissors should be kept to hand.

(Resectoscopic division of the uterine septum is further discussed in Chapter 8, and septal division with fiberoptic lasers in Chapter 9.)

The use of hysteroscopic scissors offers several advantages over the resectoscope, lasers or electrosurgery (Tables 7.2–7.4). Fluids containing electrolytes can be used and the procedure is relatively simple, easy and expedient. When approaching the area

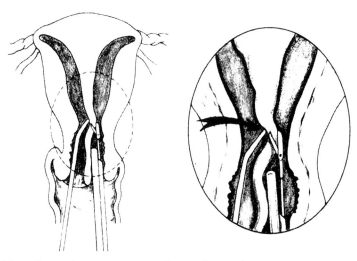

Figure 7.26 Division of a uterine septum extending to the cervix

Figure 7.27 Fenestration using semirigid scissors of a uterine septum that extends to the cervix

Figure 7.28 Septal fenestration completed

of the fundus where the myometrium begins, bleeding of small arterioles warns the hysteroscopist that the myometrium has been reached and that the operation is complete. There are, however, some disadvantages: bleeding may require coagulation; the hysteroscopic scissors are fragile and break easily or become blunt; and because no system of continuous flow for hysteros-copy has yet been perfected as with the resectoscope, if excessive fluid is used, significant absorption may occur during the procedure.

Operating electrodes mimicking bipolar systems are now in use, and while they offer the advantage of employing isotonic fluid such as saline for uterine distention, nonetheless, care should be exercised when using these devices to avoid peripheral

Figure 7.29 Completed septal fenestration, division of the remaining corporeal septum is performed

Table 7.2 Advantages and disadvantages of the use of hysteroscopic scissors

Advantages	Disadvantages
Relatively simple	Scissors become dull easily
Quick	Bleeding if not in midline
More applicable to thin septa	Possible perforation
Media with electrolytes	No washing effect unless double-channel hysteroscope used
No energy sources required	Thick septa more difficult to divide

Table 7.3 Advantages and disadvantages of the resectoscope for uterine septum

Advantages	Disadvantages
No significant bleeding	Electrosurgery required (monopolar)
Cuts quickly and easily	Possible peripheral endometrial coagulation
Washing of uterine cavity	Landmarks of myometrium lost
Excellent visibility	Fluids without electrolytes
Advantageous for broad septa	Requires proficiency with resectoscope

Table 7.4 Advantages and disadvantages of fiberoptic lasers for treatment of uterine septum

Advantages	Disadvantages
No significant bleeding	Expensive
Cuts well	Requires special protective glasses
Easy manipulation	Possible lateral scattering
Requires fluids with electrolytes	Requires special maintenance and assistance (laser safety officer)
Tedious due to size of fiber	

Table 7.5 Comparison of different methods of hysteroscopic metroplasty

Feature	Scissors	Resectoscope	Fiber lasers
Simplicity	+ +	+	+
Speed	+ + +	+ +	+
Hemostasis	+	+ + +	+ + +
Applicable to all septa	+ +	+	+ +
Evaluation of juxtaposed myometrium	+ + +	+	+
Cost	+	+ +	+ + +
Possible perforation	+	+ +	+ +
Required skill	+ + +	+ + +	+ + +
Fluid overload	+	+ +	+ +

damage to the surrounding endometrium by electrosurgical scattering.

Because it is a relatively simple procedure and avoids unnecessary damage to the surrounding endometrium, the hysteroscopic method of dividing the uterine septum with scissors continues to be the preferred method for treating this condition (Table 7.5). The reproductive outcome following hysteroscopic treatment of a symptomatic septate uterus has equaled and even surpassed the results obtained with traditional abdominal metroplasty, with a more than 85–90% rate of viable pregnancies. The patient is spared a laparotomy and hysterotomy, thereby eliminating the potential for pelvic adhesions as well as the associated pain, disability and expense. Patients treated hysteroscopically need to wait for only 4 weeks following the procedure before attempting conception, and Cesarean section is not mandatory should pregnancy be carried to term.

Practical considerations in the treatment of septa

Laparoscopy can be performed with a 5 mm laparoscope to monitor the hysteroscopic surgery. The pelvic cavity, uterus, ovaries and Fallopian tubes are systematically observed and the light of the laparoscope dimmed to allow hysteroscopic light translucency through the uterine wall.

In general, semirigid hysteroscopic scissors are sufficient to divide thin septa. For thick and broad septa, the resectoscope fitted with a thin cutting electrode is useful, as this type of electrode can reach the lateral portions of the septum to avoid bleeding. A blend of outputs made up of 80–90 W of cutting (unmodulated) output and 30–40 W of coagulating (modulated) output can be used.

On completion of septal division, the intrauterine pressure can be decreased slightly so that bleeding can be selectively coagulated before the procedure is terminated.

INTRAUTERINE ADHESIONS

The early follicular phase of the menstrual cycle is chosen in menstruating patients who demonstrate intrauterine adhesions on hysterosalpingography (Figure 7.30). Depending on the extent of uterine cavity occlusion shown by the hysterosalpingogram, laparoscopy is used concomitantly

Figure 7.30 Hysterosalpingogram showing extensive central intrauterine adhesions

Figure 7.31 Hysteroscopic division of intrauterine adhesions using semirigid scissors

in patients who demonstrate extensive uterine cavity involvement or tubal occlusion. An operative hysteroscope and semirigid hysteroscopic scissors are used to divide these adhesions (Figure 7.31). In many of these patients, the endometrium has been traumatized; therefore, additional trauma or damage due to electrosurgery and laser is avoided by using mechanical hysteroscopic scissors. Fluids containing electrolytes, specifically, normal saline, dextrose 5% in 50% saline or Ringer's lactate, are preferred for uterine distention. When laparoscopy is performed, tubal patency is evaluated by injecting indigocarmine dye transcervically. Depending on the extent of uterine cavity occlusion, an intrauterine splint is left in the uterus to keep the uterine walls separated. An indwelling catheter (number 8) with a trimmed tip is placed in the uterus with 3–3.5 ml of saline solution in the balloon and left in place for 1 week.

Prophylactic antibiotics are used both during and after the procedure particularly when splints are left in place. Cephazolin 1 g is given intravenously during the proce-

dure, followed by cephalexin 500 mg four times a day orally, or doxycycline 100 mg intravenously and 100 mg twice daily orally for 1 week until the splint is removed. To aid in the rapid re-epithelization of the uterine cavity, conjugated estrogens are prescribed. Oral Premarin® 2.5 mg twice daily is given for 30–40 days, adding terminal medroxyprogesterone acetate (Provera®) 10 mg once a day orally for the last 6–10 days of the artificial cycle to induce withdrawal bleeding. At the conclusion of the hormonal treatment and once withdrawal bleeding ceases, a hysterosalpingogram is performed to assess uterine cavity normalcy.

Normal menstruation has been re-established in over 90% of patients treated for intrauterine adhesions, but the reproductive outcome is related to the severity of the disease. The overall pregnancy rate of 60–70% correlates the extent of intrauterine cavity occlusion and adhesion composition with the reproductive outcome; the more extensive and thicker are the adhesions, the poorer is the prognosis. Valle and Sciarra reported that, in 187 patients treated hysteroscopically,

Figure 7.32 Rugged aspect of uterine cavity immediately after lysis of adhesions

Figure 7.33 Division of thick fibrous adhesions

the removal of mild filmy adhesions gave the best results, with 35 (81%) of 43 patients achieving term pregnancies; in 97 moderate cases of intramuscular adhesions, 64 (66%) term pregnancies occurred, but in 47 severe cases of connective-tissue adhesions, there were only 15 (32%) term pregnancies. Overall, restoration of normal menses occurred in 90% of patients and a term pregnancy was achieved in 80%.

Other methods of treating intrauterine adhesions include the use of a resectoscope or fiberoptic lasers (Figures 7.31–7.34), although special precautions are needed when using these techniques to avoid unnecessary damage to the already compromised endometrium. When using the resectoscope, only fine electrodes should be used and the adhesions selectively divided to avoid contact with the surrounding endometrium. Similar precautions apply with the use of vaporizing electrodes. When using lasers, only sculpted fibers with thin conical tips should be selected.

The use of hysteroscopy in the treatment of intrauterine adhesions has

Figure 7.34 Remaining fibrous stumps in the uterine wall are trimmed with biopsy forceps

markedly improved the management of these patients by identifying the type of adhesions present and allowing the selective division of adhesions atraumatically without further damage to the remaining endometrium. The reproductive outcome is better than with the earlier blind methods of treatment. Today, the treatment of choice for intrauterine adhesions is hysteroscopic division.

Results of treatment of adhesions

The results of treatment of adhesions obtained with hysteroscopy are related to the type of adhesions found. When adhesions are filmy and focal, the reproductive outcome is over 90%. For fibromuscular and thick adhesions producing moderate occlusion of the uterine cavity, the reproductive outcome is 70%; in patients with thick connective adhesions or total uterine cavity occlusion, the reproductive outcome drops to 25–30%. Therefore, an increased awareness of the possibility of intrauterine adhesions following postpartum or postabortal curettage or trauma to the uterine cavity will enhance early diagnosis by hysterosalpingography to evaluate those patients who develop menstrual abnormalities following such trauma to the endometrium.

Practical considerations in the treatment of intrauterine adhesions

The hysterosalpingogram is an important diagnostic adjunct for determining the extent of uterine cavity occlusion, and the condition of the cornual areas and Fallopian tubes. Unless total uterine cavity occlusion occurs, the hysterosalpingogram should be displayed in the operating suite to allow the physician to be aware of the uterine cavity distortion while treating these adhesions.

In general, semirigid hysteroscopic scissors are useful for selectively and systematically dividing these adhesions. Sculpted or extruded fiberoptic lasers with sharp tips may also be used. When electrosurgery is chosen, sharp electrodes can be directed through the operative channel of a continuous-flow hysteroscope to divide the adhesions. The resectoscope is not practical for treating these conditions; the available electrodes do not have tips sharp enough to divide precisely the adhesions without further damage to peripheral areas of already damaged endometrium.

Patients treated hysteroscopically for moderate or severe adhesions require a follow-up hysterosalpingogram on completion of hormonal treatment to evaluate the uterine cavity.

LOST OR MISPLACED INTRAUTERINE DEVICES

Although the use of intrauterine devices (IUDs) in the USA has markedly decreased, devices such as the Cu-T®, Progestasert® IUD and Mirena IUD are still in use. Unnecessary irradiation may occur when X-rays are used routinely for diagnostic purposes. Potentially traumatic manipulations are often performed in an attempt to remove the devices. In the majority of patients with missing IUDs, the IUD in fact remains in the uterine cavity, usually with the filaments curled up in the fundus of the uterus (Figures 7.35–7.37).

Hysteroscopy is particularly useful not only to detect the IUD and rule out translocation, but also to aid in its atraumatic removal.

After the IUD is located, an operative hysteroscope with grasping forceps is used to grasp either the strings or the IUD itself to retrieve the IUD. This procedure requires only local anesthesia and can easily be performed in an outpatient ambulatory surgical unit or, if the instrumentation is available, in the office.

When the IUD is not visualized in the uterine cavity, a single flat-plate X-ray of the abdomen and pelvis is required to rule out translocation.

Figure 7.35 Copper-7 intrauterine device (IUD) with its filament curled up in the uterine cavity

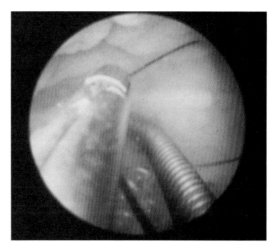

Figure 7.36 Hysteroscopic retrieval of misplaced copper-7 IUD

Figure 7.37 This copper-7 IUD is deeply embedded in the uterine wall

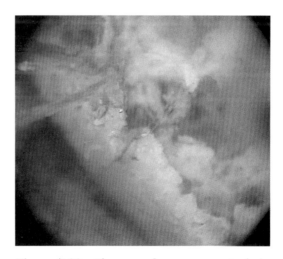

Figure 7.38 Plaques of osseous metaplasia found at hysteroscopy

Another condition amenable to hysteroscopic treatment is the formation of osseous metaplasia and calcifications that can occur following an abortion, particularly in the second trimester. The systematic removal of these plaques is accomplished under direct vision in order to re-establish normalcy to the uterine cavity and restore fertility (Figures 7.38 and 7.39).

ENDOMETRIAL ABLATION

Abnormal uterine bleeding is a frequent problem that requires appropriate evaluation and treatment. When the bleeding is due to an organic uterine pathology, the condition must be treated by removing the offending lesion or, when this is not possible or indicated, by performing a hysterectomy.

Figure 7.39 Hysteroscopic removal of osseous metaplastic plaques

In the absence of organic pathology, abnormal bleeding from the uterus is usually due to either hormonal imbalances or local factors interfering with appropriate hemostasis. Most patients with this type of dysfunctional bleeding respond to treatment with progesterone, a combination of estrogens and progesterone or non-steroidal anti-inflammatory agents and, for those patients with anovulatory cycles who are interested in fertility, treatment for anovulation.

There is a group of patients, however, who do not respond to hormonal therapy and require hysterectomy to treat abnormal bleeding. While a hysterectomy indeed relieves the symptoms, such major surgery causes additional disability, significant expense and inconvenience to the patient. In addition, there are patients at risk of major surgery because of other medical conditions such as coagulopathies, pulmonary and renal problems, and morbid obesity. For these patients, an alternative treatment to hysterectomy is desirable.

Endometrial ablation was introduced to treat abnormal uterine bleeding of dysfunc-tional origin as an alternative to hysterectomy. Many patients object to hysterectomy unless it is absolutely necessary and enthusiastically choose endometrial ablation. These patients should be assessed to rule out malignant or premalignant conditions of the endometrium and other organic pathology. A hormonal preparation is also necessary to produce thinning of the endometrium to improve the chances of destroying the whole of the endometrium, including the basal layer and the superficial (2–3 mm) layer of the myometrium. To accomplish this, fiberoptic lasers or electrosurgery to resect or coagulate the lining of the uterus can be used (Table 7.6). Danazol or GnRH analog should then be given for 6–8 weeks.

Laser endometrial ablation

This requires a laser that transmits through fluids, is attracted and absorbed by pigments and the purplish color of vascularized endometrium, and penetrates deeply (4–5 mm) into tissue (Table 7.6). Such a laser is the Nd : YAG laser which uses a bare fiber (600–800 µm) with 55–65 W of power. To thin the endometrium and make the surface more uniform, it is important to treat these patients hormonally prior to the procedure, using danazol 800 mg/day for 6 weeks or a Gn-RH analog, such as depot Lupron 3.75 mg intramuscularly, preferably in two separate injections 1 month apart, to accomplish complete atrophy of the endometrium.

The patient is placed in a dorsal lithotomy position and regional or general anesthesia is used. Because no electrical conduction is involved, the fluids used to distend the uterine cavity should contain electrolytes, for example normal saline,

Table 7.6 Comparison of different methods for performing endometrial ablation according to complications

Feature	Laser	Roller-ball/bar	Resection
Uterine perforation	++	+	+++
Fluid overload		+	+++
contact	+++		
non-contact	+		
combination	++		
Bleeding		+	+++
contact	+++		
non-contact	+		
combination	++		
Injury to adjacent organs	++	+	+++
Coagulation necrosis of uterine wall	+	+	–
Recurrent abnormal bleeding	+	++	++
Pregnancy	+	+	+
Eventual hysterectomy	+	+	+

dextrose 5% in 50% saline or Ringer's lactate. Ideally, the operative hysteroscope should have a continuous-flow capacity to cleanse the uterine cavity and permit measurement of the recovered fluid. Three different techniques can be used when performing endometrial ablation with the Nd : YAG laser.

Dragging or touching

The bare fiber is dragged across the endometrial surface (Figures 7.40 and 7.41). To ensure that all of the tissue is treated, it is important to treat surfaces systematically, beginning at the uterotubal cornua – the most difficult and potentially dangerous site because of the thinness of the uterine wall – followed by the fundal area. Once this is accomplished, treatment can then extend to the anterior, lateral and posterior walls as far as the internal os. To avoid cervical stenosis, care should be taken not to treat the endocervical tissue. The fiber should always be dragged towards the operator.

Blanching

The blanching or non-contact technique differs from dragging in that the fiber is held about 1–2 mm from the tissue surface and fired (see Figures 7.42 and 7.43). The treated area is thus blanched but, as no furrows or sulci are made, the chances of fluid intravasation are decreased as no additional vascular sinuses are opened. Bleeding does not occur as the treatment is strictly by coagulation. However, as it is difficult to keep track of the areas treated owing to the lack of clear differentiation with blanching, in contrast to the dark brown areas left by dragging, it is important to draw lines of demarcation or quadrants in the uterine cavity to avoid leaving behind untreated areas. The technique is similar to dragging in terms of the order in which different areas of endometrium are treated.

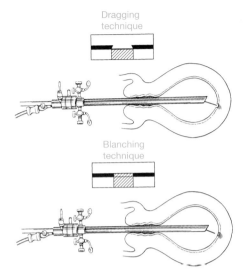

Figure 7.40 Dragging and blanching techniques for endometrial ablation

Figure 7.41 Hysteroscopic view of dragging technique for endometrial ablation

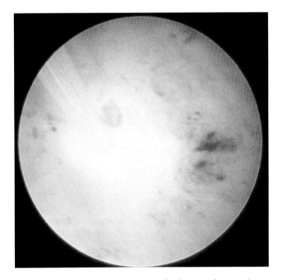

Figure 7.42 Appearance of the endometrium with application of the blanching technique

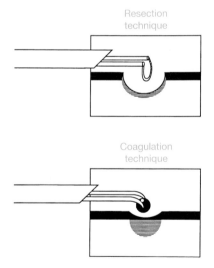

Figure 7.43 Endometrial ablation by resection compared with coagulation using a resectoscope

Dragging and blanching in combination

Both techniques can be applied, using the non-contact method in the cornual areas and the dragging technique in the rest of the endometrial cavity. This is the most commonly used method of endometrial ablation by laser.

Electrosurgical endometrial ablation

As an alternative to the laser method, electrosurgery can be used to accomplish endometrial ablation by endometrial resection with a loop electrode or coagulation with a rollerball/bar electrode.

Table 7.7 Comparison of neodymium : yttrium–aluminum–garnet (Nd : YAG) laser and electrosurgery for endometrial ablation

Feature	Nd : YAG laser	Electrosurgery
Cost of equipment	Expensive	Moderate
Ancillary help	Important	Minimal
Duration of procedure	+++	+
Cure rate	Excellent	Excellent
Failures (bleeding)	< 5%	5–10%
Electrical conduction	–	+
Fluids with electrolytes	+	–
Simultaneous laparoscopy	–	–
Field of view	Good	Reduced
Ambulatory procedure	+	+

Figure 7.44 Coagulation using a roller-ball electrode for endometrial ablation

Figure 7.45 Endometrial ablation using a roller-bar electrode

Endometrial resection

With this method, the endometrium and superficial layer of myometrium are shaved with care to ensure that the depth of myometrial resection is 2–3 mm, to avoid perforation or excessive bleeding (Table 7.7). Because this technique is more cumbersome and dangerous at the cornual regions, most physicians prefer to do the cornual regions by coagulation (Figure 7.43).

Endometrial ablation by coagulation

Using roller-ball/bar electrodes, the endometrium can be systematically desiccated (Figures 7.44 and 7.45). Although no standard waveform or watt power is used, it is important to obtain results similar to those seen with the Nd : YAG laser. Because electrosurgery is involved, fluids devoid of electrolytes should be used, for example, glycine 1.5%, sorbitol 3%, a combination of sorbitol 2.8% and mannitol

0.5%, or mannitol 5%. A resectoscope 8–9 mm in outer diameter is used.

To avoid high voltages and erratic electrical behavior, an unmodulated or undamped 100–120-W output is preferable. Although coagulating or damped and modulated outputs can be used, they are high-voltage and produce more bubbling when used in the uterus which interferes with visualization. Additionally, a damped and modulated output is more erratic and causes excessive debris to adhere to the electrode, requiring continuous changing of the electrodes to produce uniform tissue coagulation. Studies have shown that a pure cutting or unmodulated output of about 100–120 W is sufficient to achieve endometrial destruction, including the superficial 2–3-mm layer of myometrium.

Endometrial ablation is not a hysterectomy; the patient should be carefully evaluated to confirm that bleeding is not of organic etiology. Other symptoms such as cyclical pain may represent adenomyosis. In addition, the physician and patient should have realistic expectations as the goal of this procedure is not to obtain amenorrhea, but to treat abnormal uterine bleeding.

Results of endometrial ablation

When the proposed guidelines of proper selection and preparation of patients are followed, patients can expect an 85–90% resolution of abnormal bleeding. Patients who fail to respond to the procedure may attempt a second endometrial ablation, if so desired, as the results may improve on the second attempt. It is important to rule out organic conditions such as myomas and/or adenomyosis that may increase the possibility of failure.

While patients at risk of a hysterectomy because of medical conditions benefit most from endometrial ablation, other patients with dysfunctional uterine bleeding unresponsive to hormonal treatment may also benefit from this alternative should they object to hysterectomy. They should be made aware of the requirements and limitations inherent with this approach. (For more details on resectoscopic endometrial ablation, see Chapter 8.)

Although many new techniques of so-called 'global' endometrial ablation have been introduced, for the most part all of them are carried out blindly and not guided visually, with the exception of the hydrothermal method that permits the introduction of heated fluid through a hysteroscopic channel under direct vision. Nonetheless, the same rules as for any method of endometrial ablation apply, such as good patient selection, preparation of the patient with complete uterine evaluation to rule out organic pathology or malignant or premalignant endometrial lesions, and continued follow-up. All of the new methods of endometrial ablation that have appeared lately must measure up in their results to the standard laser and electrosurgical endometrial ablation procedures.

TUBAL CANNULATION

Tubal occlusion at the cornual regions can be detected during hysterosalpingography in the evaluation of infertile patients (Table 7.8). Because around 20–30% of these occlusions may be due to temporary spasm, these patients require additional evaluation to rule out such a possibility. Various pharmacological agents, for example, glucagon, ixosuprine

Table 7.8   Evaluation of tubal cornual occlusion

Rules out tubal spasm (laparoscopy)
Diagnoses/treats pelvic adhesions, endometriosis, etc.
Rules out distal tubal occlusion
Most infertile patients require laparoscopy
Requires fluoroscopic cannulation if previous laparoscopy normal or contraindicated
If fluoroscopic cannulation fails, proceed with hysteroscopic cannulation (more accurate)

and sedatives, have been used to reduce spasm, but none has been successful in eliminating this problem. Therefore, laparoscopy under general anesthesia has been the method of choice. When laparoscopy demonstrates a true tubal cornual occlusion, the patient becomes a candidate for microsurgery to remove the occluded segments and subsequent anastomosis (Figure 7.46). Because frequently the tubal segments removed do not demonstrate true occlusion, the question arises as to the origin of the occlusion. In one series where tubal segments were subjected to histopathological evaluation, it was found that, in more than half of the patients, the occlusion was due to tenacious mucus plugs or amorphous proteinaceous material that could be dislodged by probing. This finding confirmed previous clinical observations and prompted the use of tubal cannulation to evaluate and treat these patients.

While hysteroscopic tubal cannulation began in the early 1920s with attempts to occlude the Fallopian tubes transcervically by coagulation for sterilization, it was not until the 1960s that tubal cannulation was introduced by Menken, and perfected by Quinones in the early 1970s. Borrowing from the experience obtained with vascular cannulation and angioplastic procedures, tubal cannulation was initiated by radiologists in the early 1980s with the soft, flexible, coaxial catheters used in angiographic procedures. This method proved to be feasible, effective and reproducible. Because a

significant number of patients who have cornual occlusions may also harbor pelvic pathology such as pelvic adhesions, endometriosis or distal tubal occlusion, the need for laparoscopy encouraged physicians to use the hysteroscope as a more precise and direct method of cannulating the Fallopian tubes with concomitant laparoscopy not only to evaluate the pelvis, ovaries and Fallopian tubes, but also to rule out patients who have spasm rather than tubal occlusion (Table 7.9).

The hysteroscopic method requires coaxial catheters similar to those used during fluoroscopic procedures. A 3-Fr catheter inserted into a 5-Fr catheter is the most commonly used coaxial system (Figure 7.47). A soft guidewire that fits inside the 3-Fr catheter and measures no more than 0.5 mm in diameter is used to find the tubal openings. The coaxial catheters are inserted into the operating channel of an operative hysteroscope (Figure 7.48).

Most physicians use low-viscosity fluids such as normal saline, dextrose 5% in 50% saline solution or Ringer's lactate. The coaxial catheters are directed towards the uterotubal cornua and the soft guidewire used to probe the tubal opening without forcing its entrance. The distal portion of the guidewire can be stiffened as the catheters are slid forward and, should the inner catheter and soft wire become too stiff, the catheters can be withdrawn to restore flexibility. Once the guidewire has

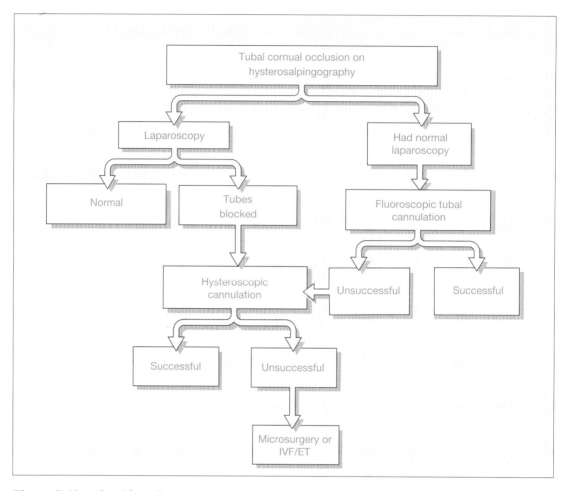

Figure 7.46 Algorithm for evaluation and treatment of tubal occlusion. IVF/ET, *in vitro* fertilization/embryo transfer

Table 7.9 Comparison of hysteroscopic and fluoroscopic tubal cannulation techniques

Feature	Hysteroscopy (laparoscopy)	Fluoroscopy
Rule out spasm	+	−
Rule out pelvic adhesions	+	−
Diagnosis/treatment of distal tubal occlusion	+	−
Accuracy	++	+
Invasive (relatively)	++	+
Radiation exposure	−	+
Cost	++	+
Time	++	+
Expertise	+	+
General anesthesia	+	−

Figure 7.47 A 3-Fr catheter inserted into a 5-Fr catheter, with a flexible guidewire in place, is the most commonly used coaxial system

Figure 7.48 Coaxial catheter and guidewire deflected by the lever of the hysteroscope

passed through the cornual region, the 3-Fr catheter is slid over the guidewire, which is fixed distally. When the first portion of the isthmic tube is reached, the guidewire guide is removed and indigo–carmine dye injected through the catheter to ascertain tubal patency as assessed by concomitant laparoscopy. The same procedure is performed in the opposite tube should bilateral obstruction be present.

When there is resistance to passing the guidewire and catheter into the Fallopian tube, the operation should be aborted as this indicates that the tube has a fibrotic occlusion rather than a mucous or proteinaceous plug that can be dislodged by cannulation. These patients should be offered either microsurgical treatment or *in vitro* fertilization.

Results of tubal cannulation

The results of hysteroscopic tubal cannulation are promising: rates of tubal recanalization range from 70 to 90%; and intrauterine pregnancy rates range from 45

to 50%. Nevertheless, the 20–30% reocclusion rate and 8% rate of ectopic pregnancy should be borne in mind.

Hysteroscopic tubal cannulation (Figures 7.49 and 7.50) has been found to be an excellent method of selecting those patients who may benefit most from microsurgery, and is the best initial diagnostic method and an excellent therapeutic alternative for patients with non-fibrotic tubal obstructions. Because patients with tubal occlusions may have concomitant pelvic pathology, such as adhesions and/or endometriosis, these conditions may also be evaluated and treated during laparoscopy.

Practical considerations in tubal cannulation

Rigid operative hysteroscopes are best used with coaxial Novy catheters with a 3-Fr catheter inserted within a 5-Fr catheter and an intraluminal guidewire < 0.5 mm in diameter. Should a flexible 5-mm operative hysteroscope be selected, the Katayama 3-Fr catheter with its guidewire should be

Figure 7.49 Hysteroscopic tubal cannulation using a flexible (left) and rigid (right) hysteroscope

Figure 7.50 Right tubal cannulation showing passing of indigo–carmine injected through catheter

Figure 7.51 Katayama 3-Fr catheter with guidewire for use with flexible hysteroscopes (Cook Ob/Gyn)

used (Figure 7.50). No additional coaxial catheters are needed as these 60-cm catheters can be inserted directly into the 2 mm operative channel and selectively bent or steered to a position in apposition to the tubal opening (Figure 7.51). A similar method is followed when using small-caliber hysterscopes with continuous-flow systems and 5-Fr operative channels (Figure 7.52).

Laparoscopy is performed to evaluate the pelvis and rule out additional pathology such as adhesions, endometriosis and/or distal tubal occlusion. Should these types of pathology be found, they can be treated directly under laparoscopic control. If tubal distal occlusion is diagnosed, the tubal cannulation procedure should be aborted, as these patients will benefit more from the new assisted-reproduction technologies,

Figure 7.52 A 3-Fr catheter in place in the operating channel of a flexible hysteroscope

such as *in vitro* fertilization and embryo transfer, than from treatment of bipolar or double tubal occlusion.

Laparoscopy is also performed to rule out tubal spasm, and indigo–carmine dye is injected transcervically to assess tubal patency and confirm cornual occlusion. Although some physicians prefer to perform tubal cannulation under fluoroscopy, there are drawbacks to this approach. Tubal spasm cannot be ruled out and, therefore, some patients may undergo tubal cannulation unnecessarily. Tubal and peritoneal pathology cannot be evaluated without laparoscopy, particularly tubal and/or ovarian adhesions, endometriosis and distal tubal occlusion. Should fluoroscopic cannulation fail, these patients should be offered hysteroscopic tubal cannulation before deciding on microsurgery for tubal reconstruction.

Because manipulation of the Fallopian tube is involved, it is prudent to give these patients prophylactic broad-spectrum antibiotics, such as cephalosporins or doxycycline, to prevent tubal infection. A subsequent hysterosalpingogram will be necessary if the patient fails to conceive within 8–9 months following the operation.

During these procedures, as with any other hysteroscopic therapeutic procedure, a video system is mandatory as it increases the awareness of the assisting physicians and permits sharing the operation with the operating team.

HYSTEROSCOPIC TUBAL STERILIZATION

For years, the need to simplify tubal sterilization by avoiding general anesthesia, the morbidity associated with incisions, and prolonged recovery periods, have motivated physicians to look for a transcervical method of sterilization. This quest, however, has been elusive, despite enormous interest in the early 1970s. Recently, a new method of transcervical tubal sterilization called the ESSURE™ permanent contraceptive system was developed by the California-based company, Conceptus, Inc. The ESSURE device underwent extensive evaluation *in vivo* and *in vitro* to determine acute and chronic anchoring as well as complete tubal occlusion to resolve problems with the original transcervical sterilization methods, such as difficulty in securing tubal devices *in situ* and consistent occlusion of the Fallopian tubes.

Histological response to the ESSURE microinsert was characteristic of the histological response observed with the use of polyethylene terephthalate (PET) fibers in other anatomical sites – specifically, a strong fibrous tissue response extending into the space of the device was viewed in the inner and outer coils of the ESSURE microinsert. The histological response consisted of both loose and dense fibrosis and smooth muscle cells migrating from the Fallopian tube wall into the space between the inner and the outer coil. This response was consistent throughout 3 months of wearing (Figures 7.53–7.56).

Technique of insertion and deployment

The patient is placed in the dorsal lithotomy position and the vaginal area and cervix cleansed with an antiseptic solution. A paracervical block is performed with a local anesthetic. Any local anesthetic can be used to perform the paracervical block, nonetheless, because of its low toxicity, an ester-type of anesthetic is preferable, such as chloroprocaine (Nesacaine) 1% solution, injecting 4-6 ml of the solution superficially at the base of each uterosacral ligament. A small amount of anesthetic (0.5 ml) can also be applied on the anterior lip of the cervix to place the tenaculum without discomfort to the patient.

A small-caliber, 3.9–5.9 mm outer diameter hysteroscope with a continuous-flow system and 5-Fr operative channel is used. The tenaculum is optional, placed on the anterior lip of the cervix, and hysteroscopy performed without previous cervical dilatation. Low-viscosity fluids such as normal saline are preferable when using the hysteroscopic method with continuous-flow system. The normal saline is warmed to room temperature to avoid discomfort to the patient by cooling. These procedures are best performed with a video camera to share with the patient the steps in performing the sterilization. The uterine cavity is evaluated and both tubal openings are observed. The ESSURE microinsert is set through the 5-Fr operative channel of the hysteroscope and gently guided into the tubal opening until the dark circle of the outer catheter comes into view, simplifying deployment. The wheel in the handle is activated until a stop occurs, showing the microinsert in the tubal lumen still not deployed and housed in the catheter. A metal notch marker comes into view signifying good placement, and by pressing the small button in the handle, the microinsert is deployed. Further turning of the wheel in the handle will demonstrate the anchoring of the microinsert by expansion of the spring outer coils. Several counterclockwise turns finally detach the delivery system, and the microinsert proximal end is evaluated by hysteroscopy to ensure that 5–10 mm (5–10 coils) of trailing microinsert are in the uterine cavity. The same procedure is performed in the opposite Fallopian tube.

Clinical evaluation prior to pre-marketing approval in women with documented fertility who selected investigational hysteroscopic permanent contraception with ESSURE microinserts demonstrated bilateral occlusion in 96%. At 6 months' follow-up, bilateral occlusion was demonstrated in all patients. The ESSURE method was approved by the FDA on November 4, 2002. Because it is a truly ambulatory office procedure, the ESSURE method of contraception promises to be an excellent alternative for women by decreasing morbidity, cost and inconvenience to the patient.

PRACTICAL CONSIDERATIONS IN OPERATIVE HYSTEROSCOPY

The operative hysteroscope should be manipulated with care while maintaining the foreoblique orientation of the instrument. Movements are delicate and the endoscope can be turned clockwise or counterclockwise

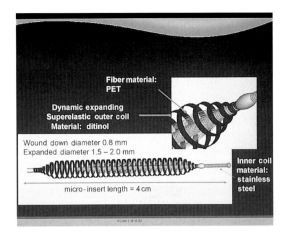

Figure 7.53 Diagram of ESSURE™ microinsert (Conceptus, Inc.)

Figure 7.54 Histological section at intramural–isthmic region of a Fallopian tube fitted with ESSURE microinsert (after 12 weeks of wearing)

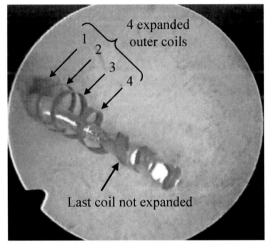

Figure 7.55 ESSURE microinsert in place with trailing tail in uterine cavity

Figure 7.56 Hysterosalpingogram 3 months after placement of ESSURE device shows complete tubal occlusion

to see either side of the uterus. Manipulation of the operative instruments, particularly those of the semirigid type, should be performed with care to avoid excessive bending, as these instruments are easily broken. If bleeding occurs, and a continuous-flow system does not clear the view, a polyethylene catheter 2.5 mm in outer diameter and 1.7 mm in inner diameter can be introduced

to evacuate any blood clots or debris that may obscure the view. It is important to use this maneuver even before uterine distention begins, as dilatation of the cervix usually causes bleeding that may obscure the view when injecting fluids.

Video cameras, when used, must not be turned; only the hysteroscope should rotate. The camera is kept in place with one hand to avoid losing the orientation of the field. If the view is clouded, the lenses as well as the ocular part of the hysteroscope and the camera lens should be removed and cleaned with a dry sponge. Clouding may be due to moisture particularly as the procedure progresses, as fluid may enter the interface and fog the lenses. This phenomenon also occurs frequently when the camera is housed in a plastic hood to avoid contamination. The camera should be adapted to the hysteroscope before the hysteroscope is introduced into the uterus; the colors should be selected while looking at a white cloth, and the image should be focused before inserting the scope. All operating instruments should be placed on the table, readily available for immediate use.

The use of hysteroscopy as a therapeutic tool involves a variety of conditions that can best be treated by this approach. The feasibility of treating intrauterine lesions with minimal invasion brings hysteroscopy to its maximum potential in gynecology.

SELECTED BIBLIOGRAPHY

Baggish MS, Baltoyannis P. New techniques for laser ablation of the endometrium in high risk patients. *Am J Obstet Gynecol* 1988;159:287

Baggish MS, Sze EHM, Morgan G. Hysteroscopic treatment of symptomatic submucous myomata uteri with the Nd:YAG laser. *J Gynecol Surg* 1989;5:27

Baggish MS, Sze EHM, Rosenzweig BA, et al. Direct hysteroscopic observation to document the reasons for abnormal uterine bleeding secondary to submucous myoma. *J Gynecol Surg* 1989;5:149

Buttram VC, Gibbons WE. Mullerian anomalies: a proposed classification (an analysis of 44 cases). *Fertil Steril* 1979;32:40

Candiani GB, Vercellini P, Fedele L, *et al*. Repair of the uterine cavity after hysteroscopic septal incision. *Fertil Steril* 1990;54:991

Cohen L, Valle RF. Role of vaginal sonography and hysterosonography in the endoscopic treatment of uterine myomas. *Fertil Steril* 2000;73:1997–2004

Confino E, Tur-Kaspa I, DeCherney A, et al. Transcervical balloon tuboplasty. A multi-center study. *J Am Med Assoc* 1990;264:2079

Daly DC, Walters CA, Soto-Albors CE, Riddick DH. Hysteroscopic metroplasty: surgical technique and obstetric outcome. *Fertil Steril* 1983;39:623

Daly DC, Tohan N, Walters C, Riddick DH. Hysteroscopic resection of the uterine septum in the presence of a septate cervix. *Fertil Steril* 1983;39:560

DeCherney AH, Polan ML. Hysteroscopic management of intrauterine adhesions and intractable uterine bleeding. *Obstet Gynecol* 1983;61:392

DeCherney AH, Russell JB, Graebe RA, Polan ML. Resectoscopic management of mullerian fusion defects. *Fertil Steril* 1986;45:726

Derman SG, Rehnstrom J, Neuwirth RS. The long-term effectiveness of hysteroscopic treatment of menorrhagia and leiomyomas. *Obstet Gynecol* 1991;77:591

Donnez J, Schours B, Gillerot S, et al. Treatment of uterine fibroids with implants of gonadotropin-releasing hormone agonist: assessment of hysterography. *Fertil Steril* 1989;51:947

Fedele L, Arcaini L, Parazzini F, et al. Reproductive prognosis after hysteroscopic metroplasty in 102 women: life-table analysis. *Fertil Steril* 1993;59:768

Friedman A, Defazio J, DeCherney AH. Severe obstetric complications following hysteroscopic lysis of adhesions. *Obstet Gynecol* 1986;67:864

Garry R. Hysteroscopic alternatives to hysterectomy. *Br J Obstet Gynaecol* 1990;97:199

Gimpelson RJ. Hysteroscopic Nd:YAG ablation of the endometrium. *J Reprod Med* 1988;38:872

Goldrath MH, Fuller TA, Segal S. Laser photovaporization of the endometrium for the treatment of menorrhagia. *Am J Obstet Gynecol* 1981;140:14

Hassiakos DK, Zourlas PA. Transcervical division of the uterine septa. *Obstet Gynecol Surv* 1990;45:165

Klein SM, Garcia CR. Asherman's syndrome: a critique and current review. *Fertil Steril* 1973;24:722

Lin BL, Miyamoto N, Aoki R, Iwata Y. Transcervical resection of submucous myomas. *Acta Obstet Gynecol Jpn* 1986;38:1647

Loffer FD. Hysteroscopic endometrial ablation with Nd : YAG laser using a noncontact technique. *Obstet Gynecol* 1987;69:679

Loffer FD. Removal of large symptomatic intrauterine growths by the hysteroscopic resectoscope. *Obstet Gynecol* 1990;76:836

Lomano JM. Dragging technique versus blanching technique for endometrial ablation with the Nd : YAG laser in the treatment of chronic menorrhagia. *Am J Obstet Gynecol* 1988;159:152

March CM, Israel R. Gestational outcome following hysteroscopic lysis of adhesions. *Fertil Steril* 1981;36:445

Neuwirth RS, Amin HK. Excision of submucous fibroids with hysteroscopic control. *Am J Obstet Gynecol* 1976;126:95

Novy MJ, Thurmond AS, Patton P, et al. Diagnosis of cornual obstruction by transcervical fallopian tube cannulation. *Fertil Steril* 1988;50:434

Onbargi LC, Hayden R, Valle RF, Del Priore G. Effects of power and electrical current density variations in an *in vitro* endometrial ablation model. *Obstet Gynecol* 1993;82:912–18

Quinones-Guerrero R, Alvarado-Duran A, Aznar-Ramos R. Tubal catheterization: applications of a new technique. *Am J Obstet Gynecol* 1972;114:674

Rankin L, Steinberg LH. Transcervical resection of the endometrium: a review of 400 consecutive patients. *Br J Obstet Gynaecol* 1992;99:911

Rock JA, Murphy AA, Cooper WH. Resectoscopic techniques for the lysis of a class V: complete uterine septum. *Fertil Steril* 1987;48:495

Schenker JG, Margalioth EJ. Intrauterine adhesions: anupdated appraisal. *Fertil Steril* 1982;37:593

Siegler AM, Valle RF. Therapeutic hysteroscopic procedures. *Fertil Steril* 1988;50:685

Sulak PJ, Letterie GS, Coddington CC, *et al.* Histology of proximal tubal occlusion. *Fertil Steril* 1987;48:437

Thurmond AS, Novy M, Uchida BT, Rosch J. Fallopian tube obstruction: selective salpingography and recanalization. *Radiology* 1987; 163:511

Valle RF. Therapeutic hysteroscopy in infertility. *Int J Fertil* 1984;29:143

Valle RF. Clinical management of uterine factors in infertile patients. In Speroff L, ed. *Seminars in Reproductive Endocrinology*. New York: Thieme-Stratton, 1985:149–67

Valle R, Sciarra JJ. Hysteroscopic treatment of the septate uterus. *Obstet Gynecol* 1986;676:253

Valle RF, Sciarra JJ. Intrauterine adhesions: hysteroscopic diagnosis, classification, treatment, and reproductive outcome. *Am J Obstet Gynecol* 1988;158:1459

Valle RF. Hysteroscopic removal of submucous leiomyomas. *J Gynecol Surg* 1990;6:89

Valle RF. Tubal catheterization for sterilization purposes. In Gleicher N, ed. *Tubal Cannulation Procedures*. New York: Wiley-Liss, 1992:139–60

Valle RF. Rollerball endometrial ablation. In Gordon AG, ed. Endometrial Ablation. *Clin Obstet Gynecol Int Prac Res* 1995;9:229–316

Valle RF, Baggish MS. Endometrial carcinoma following endometrial ablation: high-risk factors predicting its occurrence. *Am J Obstet Gynecol* 1998;179:569–72

Valle RF. Tubal cannulation. In Siegler AM, ed. Hysteroscopy. *Obstet Gynecol Clin North Am* 1995; 223:519–40

Valle RF. Intrauterine bone formation causing infertility. *OBG Management* 1999; June :11–12

Valle RF. Hysteroscopic sterilization with the ESSURE system. In Sciarra JJ, ed. *Gynecology and Obstetrics. Fertility Regulation, Psychosomatic Problems, Infertility, Genetics*, Vol. 6, Ch. 40. New York: Lippincott-Raven, 2004:1–40

Wamsteker K, Emanuel MH, de Kruif JH. Transcervical hysteroscopic resection of submucous fibroids for abnormal uterine bleeding: results regarding the degree of intramural extension. *Obstet Gynecol* 1993;82:736

Wingo PA, Huezo CM, Rubin GL, et al. The mortality risk associated with hysterectomy. *Am J Obstet Gynecol* 1985;152:803

8

The resectoscope in gynecology

The resectoscope has been used by urologists for over half a century. It was introduced into gynecology in the early 1970s by Neuwirth to resect submucous leiomyomas. Since then, the urological resectoscope has been frequently adapted to make this instrument more applicable to gynecological procedures in the uterine cavity.

GYNECOLOGICAL RESECTOSCOPES

In general, most gynecological resectoscopes have been similarly adapted to allow the instrument to be atraumatically introduced into the uterus (Figures 8.1–8.4). The outer sheath in cross-section is round to conform to the endocervical canal anatomy; the insulating beak is shorter than that of the urological resectoscope; and the outer sheath has distal fenestrations to permit continuous flow and lavage of the uterine cavity, and to allow accurate measurement of the recovered fluid. The mechanism is the same as that of the continuous-flow resectoscope introduced by Iglesias. Most gynecological resectoscopes are 8–9 mm in outer diameter and use loop electrodes for resection, a roller-ball or roller-bar about 3–3.5 mm in length for coagulation and a curved cutting electrode for division of adhesions or thick uterine septa (Figures 8.5–8.7).

Because this instrument requires instillation of fluids and a method of recovery, special tubes are necessary, particularly if no mechanical pump is used to deliver the fluids. Large-bore or urological tubing deliv-

Figure 8.1 An assembled resectoscope with electrode in place (Storz)

Figure 8.2 An assembled 8-Fr (4 mm) resectoscope (Wolf)

Figure 8.3 An assembled resectoscope with a miniature camera attached to the ocular piece (Olympus)

Figure 8.4 Endoscopes used for uterine valuation include, from upper to lower, the diagnostic hysteroscope, operative hysteroscope with fixed scissors and resectoscope (Olympus)

Figure 8.5 Various electrodes for use with the resectoscope (Olympus)

Figure 8.6 Close-up view of distal end of bipolar resectoscope with vaporizing bulk-electrode in place (GyneCare)

Figure 8.7 Loop electrode for use with the bipolar resectoscope (GyneCare)

ers the fluids by gravity pressure from 3-l plastic bags and also collects the fluids. Because electrosurgery is involved, an electrical cord is fitted into the resectoscope; different waveforms may be used, depending on the procedure performed, and the outputs may be undamped or unmodulated for cutting or damped and modulated for coagulating, or even a combination of the two (a so-called blend mode).

Because unipolar electricity will be used, the patient should be properly grounded with an electrosurgical plate acting as the return electrode. Only fluids devoid of electrolytes, such as glycine 1.5%, sorbitol 3.5%, a combination of sorbitol 2.8% and mannitol 0.5% or mannitol 5%, should be used. Regardless of the medium, strict measurement of inflow and outflow should be maintained during the procedure and, periodically, the deficit or non-recovered fluid should be made known to the surgeon.

Recently the bipolar-like resectoscope has been introduced permitting the use of isotonic electrolytic fluid for uterine distention. However, this method also requires accurate account of non-recovered fluids to prevent fluid overload. Furthermore, because of the possibility of desalination with delayed hyponatremia due to excretion of hypertonic urine containing sodium and potassium and intravascular liberation of fluid free of electrolytes, close observation of these patients is needed when excessive fluid (more than 1 L) is not recovered.

APPLICATIONS

Although the most practical and commonly performed procedures with the resectoscope are for the removal of submucous leiomyomas and endometrial ablation, other procedures can be performed, including biopsies of focal lesions that require complete excision performed by a cutting loop (Figure 8.8), and removal of sessile polyps and/or shaving of the base of a removed polyp to avoid recurrences. During the latter, the basal layer of endometrium is also removed.

Submucous myomectomy

The resectoscope has facilitated resection of submucous leiomyomas, particularly those

Figure 8.8 Distal end of resectoscope with cutting loop in place (Storz)

which are broad-based or sessile. The resectoscope is fitted with a cutting loop and the myoma is shaved, beginning at the apex of the myoma until its attachment to the uterine wall is reached. The shavings are not removed from the uterine cavity unless they impair vision: the resectoscope is removed and the shavings retrieved with a polyp forceps or, if necessary, a large-bore plastic suction curette. On occasions, a resected shaving may stick to the loop, thereby obscuring the view; in this event, the bridge with its inner and outer sheaths is removed, cleaned and reinserted. When performing these maneuvers, it is important to remember that bleeding may ensue. Patience should therefore be exercised in that the blood clots and bleeding need to be washed away by the continuous-flow system before the resection is reinitiated. Once the myoma is removed and resection has reached the uterine wall, no attempt to dig into the tissue of the uterine wall should be made. The resection should be almost flush with the uterine wall as the remaining intramural portion will become intraluminal due to contractions of the uterine wall. When this no longer occurs, resection can cease. Prior to final removal of the resectoscope, the intrauterine pressure is slowly decreased by partially occluding the inflow, and any bleeding arterioles should be sought and selectively coagulated with the loop.

While it is easier and faster to resect these myomas using a pure or undamped cutting power output, if bleeding occurs, it will be difficult to perform coagulation unless a blend mode is used. For this reason, a blend output is preferable for myomectomy, using an 80–90 W pure cutting output and a 30–40 W coagulating output in blend-one mode (Figure 8.9).

When the patient has been properly evaluated by vaginal or fluid-enhanced sonography to rule out other leiomyomas and the intramural components of sessile myomas, the operator will then know in advance how much of the leiomyoma is intramural and how much is intraluminal. This evaluation will help to make a decision as to the approach taken to remove these myomas, and avoid the mistake of removing only the tip of the iceberg while leaving behind the greater portion. If vaginal sonography is insufficient, fluid-enhanced sonography may be helpful. Small quantities of sterile fluid are injected transcervically via catheter during vaginal sonography.

Endometrial ablation

There are three ways to perform electrosurgical endometrial ablation: by coagulation; by endometrial resection; and by a combination of coagulation and resection.

The roller-ball/bar electrode is most frequently used for coagulation or desiccation (Figures 8.10 and 8.11). Endometrial resection, including the superficial (2–3 mm) layer of myometrium is common in Europe,

Figure 8.9 Resectoscope removal of lesion for histological evaluation

but should be undertaken with caution, particularly at the cornua where the uterine wall is thinnest. For this reason, most physicians use the coagulation technique for the cornual regions and the resection technique for the rest of the endometrium. When combining the two techniques for resection of the entire uterine cavity, particularly in patients who do not respond adequately to preoperative hormonal treatment, resection of the endometrium without involving the myometrium can be performed, with coagulation applied only to the myometrial surface.

It is important to ensure hormonal preparation of these patients for uniform thinning of the endometrium before the procedure is performed. In addition, all patients should have a preoperative uterine evaluation and appropriate biopsies to rule out organic pathology, and premalignant and malignant conditions of endometrium.

Epidural and general anesthesia are the most commonly used methods, although conscious sedation may also be effective in some patients. Although resection is preferred in Europe, endometrial coagulation

Figure 8.10 Distal end of rotating continuous-flow resectoscope with ball electrode in place (Storz)

Figure 8.11 Electrode specially designed for vaporization (grooved-bar electrode) (ACMI)

or desiccation is preferred by most physicians in the USA because it is simple, relatively safe and effective in abolishing abnormal uterine bleeding. Nonetheless, when using the roller-ball/bar electrode for coagulation, it is important to evaluate the patient preoperatively with hysteroscopy and to carry out the appropriate biopsies to rule out malignant or premalignant lesions of the endometrium. Furthermore, these patients should receive preoperative hormonal treatment to thin the endometrium, preferably with danazol or a GnRH analog. It is not sufficient to carry out sharp or suction curettage just before ablation as this may not thin the endometrium uniformly and may leave significant amounts of tissue and debris behind, particularly in the form of endometrial stumps that hamper coagulation and render the electrodes ineffective by hindering transmission of the electrical power output to the treated tissue. Although resection may not require these precautions, routine evaluation of the endometrium with appropriate biopsies is mandatory.

Although endometrial ablation is an elective procedure requiring previous preparation, occasionally it may be needed

for acute bleeding, particularly in patients with coagulopathies. In such cases, biopsies should be performed and, if suspicious areas are found, frozen sections should be prepared before proceeding with coagulation. Thus, although bleeding patients can be treated acutely with no previous preparation, and despite the fact that these uteri usually show an atrophic endometrium, relapses may occur. It is therefore important that these patients be frequently followed-up and that they be warned of the possibility of relapse.

Occasionally, a patient receiving endometrial suppression may not be adequately suppressed. Although a thick endometrium may be found in less than 5% of these patients, superficial resection of the endometrium not including the myometrium can be performed, followed by coagulation with a roller-ball/bar electrode.

Other applications of the resectoscope are less defined or require specific modifications (Figure 8.12). These include the treatment of uterine septa with a cutting electrode and the division of intrauterine adhesions. Whereas thin septa are best treated with hysteroscopic scissors, thick broad septa benefit from the use of the

Figure 8.12 Distal end of rotating continuous-flow resectoscope with roller cutting electrode in place (Storz)

resectoscope. However, despite the fact that the electrodes currently available are not designed for this purpose, a thin electrode – preferably bent at one end – is particularly useful for treating this condition as it is able to reach the cornual extensions of broad septa and avoid damage to the endometrium. A forward-directed loop is not as efficient in reaching these areas as is the thinnest possible electrode. When using the resectoscope to divide a uterine septum, the utmost care should be exercised to maintain the symmetry of the uterine cavity during the procedure. Because electrosurgery does not permit observation of the junction between the septum and the myometrium, which may not bleed because of the electrical effect, the hysteroscopist may receive no warning that the myometrial layer has been reached. It is important, therefore, to dim the light of the laparoscope as much as possible to allow transillumination of the hysteroscopic light through the uterine wall, which may reveal to the hysteroscopist areas of possible thinning of the myometrium, thereby avoiding perforation. An alternative for monitoring these procedures is concomitant sonography.

Similarly, the resectoscope is a difficult instrument to use in the treatment of intrauterine adhesions as the currently available electrodes cannot be directed to specific areas of the uterus to selectively dissect these adhesions. Furthermore, scattering of the electrical output may damage the already compromised endometrium. For these reasons, if electrosurgery is used to divide adhesions, it is better to use needle-point electrodes guided through a hysteroscope to maximize their steerability and reduce the damage to the peripheral endometrium.

Because myomectomy with the resectoscope is a procedure that predisposes the patient to excess fluid absorption, it is important in these patients to take all the precautions necessary to avoid fluid overload (Table 8.1). An indwelling catheter should be used to measure urine output, and fluid intake and outflow, and differentials or deficits should be strictly monitored. The anesthesiologist should monitor all vital signs and pulse oximetry, and maintain careful measurement of the fluids given intravenously. In addition, regional anesthesia is preferable to general anesthesia. Finally, the electrosurgical unit should have the capability to display the type of waveform selected and the wattage requested.

BASIC TECHNIQUES IN RESECTOSCOPY

The fundamental components of a resectoscope (Figure 8.13) include: an outer sheath 8–9 mm in diameter; an inner sheath 7.5–8.5 mm in diameter; a supporting bridge for attaching the telescope and various electrodes; a telescope 4 mm in diameter with a

Table 8.1 Avoiding fluid overload during hysteroscopic myomectomy

With the anesthesiologist, discuss the complexity of the procedure, intravenous fluids, patient's risks
Consider epidural anesthesia in high-risk patients
Place indwelling catheter to monitor urine output
Keep accurate account of fluid deficit (inflow/outflow)
Look for signs of decompensation: vital signs, decreased oxygenation (pulse oximetry), hypothermia (esophageal probe) and ECG
If the deficit is > 800 ml, evaluate electrolytes (Na), status of procedures and patient's condition
Stop procedure if deficit is > 1000 ml, electrolytes (Na) decrease, there are positive signs of decompensation or extended time is needed to complete procedure

ECG, electrocardiogram

Figure 8.13 An unassembled 9-Fr resectoscope comprises, from upper to lower, the telescope, bridge, electrode and two concentric sheaths (Storz)

Figure 8.14 Distal end of a resectoscope with forward-bending cutting loop electrode in place (Storz)

12–30° angle of view; and various types of electrodes, such as loops, roller-ball/bar and a cutting knife (Figures 8.14 and 8.15).

The electrosurgical unit should display the type of waveform selected, whether undamped (cutting) or damped (coagulating). Different blends of these two waveforms and the selected wattages should also be displayed (Figures 8.16 and 8.17).

While various electrical output settings can be used for different procedures, it is important to remember the particular requirements for each of the various procedures. In general, when resecting a myoma,

Figure 8.15 Distal end of a resectoscope with knife electrode in place (Storz)

COAG1

Decaying waveform
Repeat f: 22 kHz
CF: 5.9
f: 350 kHz

COAG2

Decaying waveform
Repeat f: 30 kHz
CF: 5.6
f: 350 kHz

Pure, URO

Sine waveform
f: 350 kHz
CF: 1.5

Blend

Int. waveform
8 on/8 off
f: 350 kHz
CF: 2.3

Figure 8.16 Monopolar electrical energy waveforms (a) Cutting (unmodulated) waveform, pure for cutting and vaporization, URO (urology) for resection, and blend adding some coagulation. (b) Coagulating (modulated) waveform for desicccation. COAG1 is coagulation with little cutting capability. COAG2 is coagulation with stronger cutting capability (fulguration)

an undamped or pure cutting output may be used as it facilitates shaving of the tumor. However, on occasions, bleeding may occur and, therefore, it is useful to add a damped (coagulating) output. A useful setting is a blend of these two outputs, using 80–100 W for cutting and 30–40 W for coagulating (at blend one). The myoma is cut by activating the cutting pedal and, if coagulation is required, the appropriate output can be obtained by pressing the coagulating pedal.

While performing endometrial ablation, a specific waveform that can be measured and controlled may be selected. It is useful to remember the effects of the waveform used.

An undamped pure cutting output is optimally 100–120 W. This choice of watt power is based on experimental evidence showing that, when a cutting output of < 90 W is used, penetration is somewhat superficial (< 2 mm) and, if an output of > 120 W is used, penetration also decreases, probably due to carbonization of tissue which impedes penetration. Whenever electrical energy is used, it should preferably be of a low voltage as this appears to behave less erratically than a damped output and produces less bubbling of distending fluid in the uterus.

In contrast, a pure coagulating output of 40–50 W appears to be sufficient for 3 mm

Figure 8.17 This electrosurgical unit is capable of displaying different waveforms (Olympus)

of penetration, with the ball-electrode rolled at a uniform speed. If the watt power is increased to more than 50 W, more debris accumulates on the electrodes, requiring frequent changes to achieve the desired penetration. Furthermore, this type of high-voltage waveform also produces excessive bubbling, leading to pauses during the procedure while the excessive foam caused by the bubbles is evacuated.

It must be remembered, however, that many variables may affect the amount of tissue penetration produced by electrosurgery. Therefore, waveform and wattage, although important, are not the only criteria for adequate tissue penetration. The speed of the roller-ball/bar electrode, the size and shape of the selected electrodes and tissue impedance also play major roles.

PRACTICAL CONSIDERATIONS IN RESECTOSCOPY

The resectoscope should be assembled appropriately, ensuring that the electrodes are well fixed and secure, and that the electrical cable is in place before the electrosurgical unit is activated. It is useful to test the

electrical power before initiating the procedure by first touching the relevant tissue – the myoma, if a myomectomy is to be performed, or the uterine wall, if ablation is intended. If cervical dilatation is difficult, an obturator fitted to the assembled inner and outer cannulas may help in the initial introduction. The cervical canal should be dilated to at least the size of the resectoscope or 0.5 mm more to permit easy insertion of the resectoscope through the cervical canal. If resected tissue adheres to the loop or electrode and obstructs the view, the resectoscope and its attachments should be removed and cleaned. It is necessary to remove the assembled resectoscope for cleaning. Before removal, the running fluid should be stopped, by turning the inflow stopcock, to avoid splashing the fluid onto the floor.

On initial insertion of the resectoscope, it is important to be patient and wait until all blood clots and debris are removed by the continuous-flow system before proceeding with the operation. The dominant hand should always be used to manipulate the resectoscope while the other hand stabilizes the video camera.

The electrodes should be changed periodically, particularly if they become covered by excessive tissue or are bent. When roller-ball/bar electrodes are used, it is important to have several electrodes to hand which can be exchanged as needed. The removed electrode can be cleaned by the assistant nurse, who should remove the debris with sandpaper and appropriate cloths or sponges.

The loop electrode should not be used for myomas without the electrical output being activated, as it may be easily bent or broken. Loops can be used on soft tissue without electrosurgery for superficial shaving of a thick endometrium or a polyp.

SELECTED BIBLIOGRAPHY

Bieber EJ, Loffer FD, eds. *Gynecologic Resectoscopy.* Cambridge, MA: Blackwell Science, 1995

Cohen L, Valle RF. Role of vaginal sonography and hysterosonography in the endoscopic treatment of uterine myomas. *Fertil Steril* 2000;73:1997–2004

DeCherney AH, Russell JB, Graebe RA, Polan ML. Resectoscopic management of mullerian fusion defects. *Fertil Steril* 1986;45:726

DeCherney AH, Diamond MP, Lavy G, Polan ML. Endometrial ablation for intractable uterine bleeding: hysteroscopic resection. *Obstet Gynecol* 1987;70:668

Friedman A, Defazio J, DeCherney AH. Severe obstetric complications following hysteroscopic lysis of adhesions. *Obstet Gynecol* 1986;67:864

Hallez JP, Netter A, Cartier R. Methodical intrauterine resection. *Am J Obstet Gynecol* 1987;156:1080

Iglesias JJ, Sporer A, Gellman AC, Seebode JJ. New Iglesias resectoscope with continuous irrigation, simultaneous suction, and low intravesicle pressure. *J Urol* 1975;114:929

Kivnick S, Kanter M. Bowel injury from roller-ball ablation of the endometrium. *Obstet Gynecol* 1992;79:833

Loffer FD. Removal of large symptomatic intrauterine growths by the hysteroscopic resectoscope. *Obstet Gynecol* 1990;76:836

McCarthy JF. A new apparatus for endoscopic plastic surgery of the prostate, diathermia, and excision of vesical growths. *J Urol* 1931;26:695

McLucas B. The resectoscope in gynecologic surgery. *Female Patient* 1990;15:83

Neuwirth RS, Amin AK. Excision of submucous fibroids with hysteroscopic control. *Am J Obstet Gynecol* 1976;126:95

Rock JA, Murphy AA, Cooper WH. Resectoscopic techniques for the lysis of a class V: complete uterine septum. *Fertil Steril* 1987;48:495

Sullivan B, Kenny P, Seibel J. Hysteroscopic resection of fibroid with thermal injury to sigmoid. *Obstet Gynecol* 1992;80:546

Valle RF. Roller-ball endometrial ablation. In Gordon AG, ed. *Endometrial Ablation,* Vol. 9, *Baillière's Clinical Obstetrics and Gynecology.* London: Baillière-Tindall, 1995:299–316

Valle RF. The use of various energy modalities in hysteroscopy. In Brooks PG, Bradley LD, Cooper JM, eds. *Diagnostic and Operative Hysteroscopy.* Santa Fe Springs, CA: American Association of Gynecological Laparoscopy, 2001:85–6

Vercellini P, Vendola N, Colombo A, *et al.* Hysteroscopic metroplasty with resectoscope or microscissors for the correction of septate uterus. *Surg Gynecol Obstet* 1993;176:439

9

Laser hysteroscopy

Without doubt, the introduction of lasers into medicine has greatly facilitated many surgical procedures, particularly when used with endoscopes. Of the lasers available, the CO_2 laser has been most commonly used by gynecologists particularly in laparoscopy. The CO_2 laser is versatile and can be passed through the endoscope, thereby avoiding additional punctures in the abdomen. Its penetration is well controlled as what you see is what you get, and its shallow effects can be applied with precision without massive thermal damage to surrounding structures. However, its use requires transmission by an endoscope with built-in mirrors, and it does not coagulate vessels well nor can it be used through liquid media because of its lack of penetration in fluids. For these reasons, the CO_2 laser is not practical for hysteroscopy. Furthermore, its delivery requires a special system of mirrors to reflect the beam, making it impractical in hysteroscopy. As the uterus must be distended with fluids, if gases such as CO_2 are used, the smoke and plume cannot be evacuated without collapsing the uterine cavity.

Fortunately, fiberoptic lasers are available which use small fibers and can be activated through fluids, such as the Nd : YAG, argon and KTP-532 lasers (Table 9.1). Other lasers have recently been introduced, such as the holmium–YAG and the erbium–YAG, and are excellent coagulators able to penetrate further than the CO_2 laser. The fact that these newer lasers can be activated through the hysteroscope and permit operation through fluids makes them another useful alternative for hysteroscopic surgery.

The Nd : YAG laser has been the most commonly used laser for hysteroscopy particularly for endometrial ablation and, with the new sculpted fibers, for treatment of uterine septa and/or intrauterine adhesions. Because these lasers do not involve conduction, the uterine cavity can be distended with fluids containing electrolytes, thus adding a safety factor to prevent fluid overload, which can easily be avoided with the

Table 9.1 Physical properties of lasers used in hysteroscopic surgery

	Wavelength (nm)	Color spectrum	Power (W)	Absorption	Aiming beam
Argon	488–514	Blue-green	0–20	Hb + melanin	Argon
KTP-532	532	Green	0–40	Hb + melanin	KTP
Nd : YAG	1064	Near infrared	0–170	Tissue protein	Helium–neon

Hb, hemoglobin; KTP, potassium titanyl phosphate; Nd : YAG, neodymium : yttrium–aluminum–garnet

Table 9.2   Clinical features of lasers used in hysteroscopic surgery

	Passed through fiber	Scattering	Passes through fluids	Penetration (mm)	Coagulation	Cutting
Argon	+	+	+	1–2	+	+/–
KTP-532	+	+	+	1–2	+	+/–
Nd:YAG	+	+++	+	3–4	+++	+*

KTP, potassium titanyl phosphate; Nd:YAG, neodymium:yttrium–aluminum–garnet
* With sculpted tips

Figure 9.1   Lasers with conical (left) and ball-shaped (right) sculpted fiber tips

use of diuretics. However, because these lasers are attracted by pigment and reflected backward, the operator must wear either goggles or special filters to prevent injury to the retina. Alternatively, the continuous use of a video monitor may also avoid this hazard. The fibers most commonly used either are not coaxial or are bare fibers that transmit the coagulating effect of the Nd:YAG, penetrating about 4–5 mm in depth and, owing to the anterolateral scattering effect of this laser, forming craters in the tissue. This is a coagulating laser and is most useful for endometrial ablation. Sculpted fibers concentrate the energy of the laser, depending on the shape of the tip. A conical tip converts the laser into a light scalpel, and reduces the scattering and thermal damage while cutting, whereas a ball-shaped tip can be used for coagulation (Figure 9.1).

The argon and KTP-532 lasers are less used in gynecology. They can penetrate 1–2 mm into tissue and produce less scattering than the Nd:YAG laser (Figure 9.2). They can be used in contact with tissue or fired without touching the tissue and change their coagulating or cutting ability according to their distance from the tissue (Table 9.2).

CLINICAL APPLICATIONS

The hysteroscopic procedures most frequently performed with fiberoptic lasers are endometrial ablation and removal of pedunculated submucous leiomyomas (Figure 9.3). Endometrial ablation usually requires use of the Nd:YAG laser because of its capacity for deep coagulation

Figure 9.2 Schematic diagram comparing the depth of coagulative penetration and amount of scatter produced by various lasers

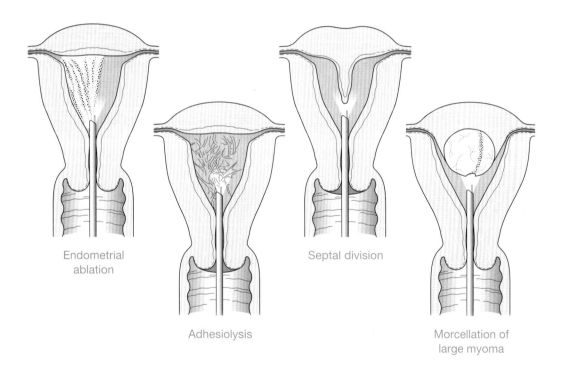

Figure 9.3 The most frequently performed hysteroscopic procedures with use of fiberoptic lasers

(4–5 mm), anterolateral scattering and penetration through fluids (Figure 9.4). Although bare fibers can be used to perform endometrial ablation, such fibers cannot be used for the more delicate operations that require controlled dissection and minimal tissue destruction, particularly peripherally, due to scattering. During removal of

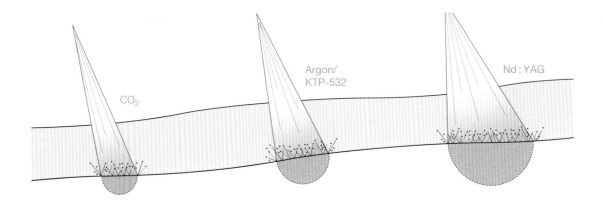

Figure 9.4   Schematic diagram showing the depth of coagulative penetration of tissue through fluid of the Nd : YAG laser compared with other lasers

pedunculated leiomyomas, the bare fiber can be used to transect the pedicle flush to the uterine wall. In addition, morcellation of large fundal myomas can be accomplished using the same technique and, occasionally, myolysis of intramural myomatous tissue can be performed with sharp sculpted fibers that can penetrate this tissue.

As regards to the treatment of polyps, an important aspect is their diagnosis. Treatment consists of blind removal of the polyp once the location has been determined, using hysteroscopic scissors or a laser for pedunculated polyps, or a resectoscope for sessile polyps. However, a laser is an expensive tool for removal of a simple polyp.

To control and concentrate the laser beam at the tip of the fiber, these fibers are manufactured in different shapes, with sharp conical tips for precise cutting and ball-shaped tips for coagulation. These lasers do not need coaxial channels for cooling, unlike the sapphire tips that are attached to the laser fiber by metallic ferrules and require continuous cooling by gases or fluids to prevent melting. However, the use of CO_2 gas to cool the sapphire tip may result in fatal gas embolism due to the high rate of flow (500–1000 ml/min) required for effective cooling. Sapphire tips should never be used in the uterine cavity, not even with cooling fluids that will mix with the distending medium, thereby increasing the intrauterine pressure and predisposing the patient to fluid overload.

Although lasers can be used to treat other conditions such as uterine septa, intrauterine adhesions and uterine polyps, their use is somewhat restricted. Polyps do not require laser treatment and the cost involved greatly outweighs the benefit. Uterine septa, particularly broad septa, can be divided with sculpted sharp laser fibers that reduce both peripheral scattering and damage to the surrounding healthy endometrium. However, this type of energy should be used with the same precautions as when dividing septa with electrosurgery using the resectoscope. The cutting and coagulating power of the laser avoids bleeding, but does not permit observation of the small arterioles that may bleed upon reaching the myometrium. Therefore, special care should be taken to avoid inadvertent penetration of the myometrial wall.

Intrauterine adhesions can also be treated, using a sharp sculpted fiber for selective division of these adhesions. However, the possibility of scatter damage to the already compromised endometrium should always be considered and only sharp sculpted fibers should be used, as required. When using lasers to treat intrauterine adhesions, particularly those located laterally at the uterotubal cornua and lateral walls, a flexible operative hysteroscope is advantageous as the laser beam can be directed perpendicularly, permitting direct and precise targeting of the laser at the areas in need of treatment. This can be more difficult when rigid endoscopes are used to manipulate these lasers.

When using lasers for operative procedures, the fluids used to distend the uterus should contain electrolytes. Because such procedures may take an extended period of time, it is important to keep an accurate account of the amount of fluid used for distention and the amount recovered to determine the deficit of unrecovered fluid. Should the amount of unrecovered fluid exceed 1500 ml, particularly if the patient has a decreased urine output, diuretics can be administered which, in conjunction with close monitoring by the anesthesiologist, should prevent fluid overload.

PRACTICAL CONSIDERATIONS IN THE USE OF LASERS

Of the various fiberoptic lasers available, the coaxial type and those requiring continuous cooling, particularly with attached sapphire tips as used in gastroenterology and/or orthopedic surgery, should not be used in the uterine cavity. The need for cooling by gases or fluids makes these lasers cumbersome to use and potentially dangerous. In particular, air, CO_2 or nitrogen to cool laser tips should never be used in the uterine cavity. Despite the coaxially injected fluids to cool sapphire tips, use of these lasers contributes to the intrauterine pressure and, thus, predisposes the patient to fluid overload by excessive absorption.

The lasers that can be used in hysteroscopy are those with sculpted or extruded tips, whether sharp and conical for cutting or rounded for coagulation. These lasers permit a more precise application of the laser beam according to requirements and do not require continuous cooling. The appropriate fiber should be selected and the power required should also be displayed by the machine. The surgeon and the assisting personnel should be provided with protective glasses or goggles and the laser should be primed or activated in a 'tongue' blade with painted colored dots before being used on the patient. The activating pedal should be pressed only by the operator and not by the assistants, and only hysteroscopes with continuous-flow systems should be used to avoid excess fluid retention. The laser should be on a stand-by setting when not in use. It is important not to drop or bend the laser fibers excessively to avoid breakage. A special sign on the door of the operating suite should be displayed warning that a laser is in use and that persons entering the room require protective goggles. Only fluids containing electrolytes should be used with lasers, with meticulous monitoring of the amounts of fluid infused and recovered undertaken by the attending circulating nurse.

While the hysteroscopic use of the laser has decreased and, for the most part, been replaced by electrosurgery, a new laser technology has been tested for the treatment of menorrhagia. The Gynelase™ 21-W diode laser fitted on a table top simplifies the cumbersome bulky lasers of the past and may offer a reasonable alternative for global endometrial ablation by employing a diffuse laser light to the entire uterine cavity. Similar precautions of selection, preparation and follow-up of these patients apply as with any other global, non-endoscopic method of endometrial ablation.

SELECTED BIBLIOGRAPHY

Baggish MS. A new laser hysteroscope for Nd–YAG endometrial ablation. *Lasers Surg Med* 1988;8:99

Baggish MS, Baltoyannis P. New techniques for laser ablation of the endometrium in high-risk patients. *Am J Obstet Gynecol* 1988;159:287

Baggish MS, Daniell J. Death caused by air embolism associated with neodymium yttrium–aluminum–garnet laser surgery and artificial sapphire tips. *Am Obstet Gynecol* 1989;161:877

Baggish MS, Sze EHM, Morgan G. Hysteroscopic treatment of symptomatic submucous myomata uteri with the Nd–YAG laser. *J Gynecol Surg* 1989;5:27

Choe JK, Baggish MS. Hysteroscopic treatment of septate uterus with neodymium–YAG laser. *Fertil Steril* 1992;57:81

Daniell JF, Osher S, Miller W. Hysteroscopic resection of uterine septi with visible light laser energy. *Colpo Gynecol Laser Surg* 1987;3:217

Diamond MP, Boyers SP, Lavy G, *et al.* Endoscopic use of the potassium-titanyl-phosphate 532 laser in gynecologic surgery. *Colpo Gynecol Laser Surg* 1987;3:213

Goldrath MH, Fuller T, Segal S. Laser photovaporization of endometrium for the treatment of menorrhagia. *Am J Obstet Gynecol* 1981;140:14

Newton RJ, Mackenzie WE, Emens MJ, Jordan JA. Division of uterine adhesions (Asherman's syndrome) with the Nd–YAG laser. *Br J Obstet Gynaecol* 1989;96:102

10

Hormonal preparation of the endometrium

The performance of hysteroscopy, particularly operative hysteroscopy, is usually timed to take place during the early follicular phase once menstruation has ceased in premenopausal patients. This is to avoid the thick luxurious endometrium encountered following ovulation (Figures 10.1 and 10.2). When the endometrium is thin and regular, hysteroscopic examination is greatly facilitated. Surgery can be accomplished without unnecessary obscuring of the view by debris, mucus or tissue floating in the distending medium. While such timing is sufficient for most hysteroscopic

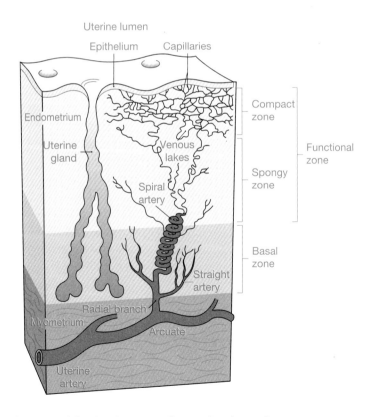

Figure 10.1   Schematic diagram of the development of normal endometrium

Figure 10.2   Schematic diagram showing changes in the endometrium during the proliferative and secretory phases of the menstrual cycle

procedures, there are two specific procedures that require additional hormonal treatment to prepare these patients for surgery, namely, endometrial ablation and (occasionally) submucous myomectomy.

During endometrial ablation, particularly when laser or electrosurgical coagulation is to be used, it is important that the endometrium be as thin (1–2 mm) and uniform as possible. This is necessary to permit the laser beam or electrical energy to penetrate and destroy not only the endometrium, including the basal layer, but also the superficial (2–3 mm) portion of the myometrium to avoid recurrences. This effect can best be obtained by treating the endometrium hormonally prior to surgery.

Several pharmacological agents cause thinning and atrophy of the endometrium, including progestogens, danazol and GnRH analogs. In the absence of these agents, both mechanical and suction curettage have been used, with less success, to

remove the functional endometrial lining prior to endometrial ablation.

PROGESTOGENS

Endometrial thinning and atrophy can be achieved with high doses of medroxyprogesterone acetate (Provera®) 20–30 mg/day, or megestrol acetate (Megace®) 20–30 mg/day for 4–6 weeks. Weekly injections of hydrosoluble progesterone 100 mg can also be given for 6 weeks. Whereas the depot forms of medroxyprogesterone acetate have been used with one to two shots 4–6 weeks apart, the results are rather unpredictable as reabsorption cannot be controlled. Although progestogens induce endometrial atrophy, they usually achieve this goal over a long period of time and high doses are necessary. Within only 4–6 weeks, there is a paradoxical response of cell decidualization, resulting in an endometrium that is thicker and more irregular and may hamper visualization. Furthermore, the side-effects of these medications, such as depression and water retention, may result in poor patient compliance.

DANAZOL

Danazol can achieve endometrial atrophy with 800 mg/day orally for 6 weeks. The endometrium is markedly decreased and, although the endometrial atrophy is more uniform and consistent than that with progestogens, some patients may not be able to tolerate the secondary androgenic side-effects.

GONADOTROPIN-RELEASING HORMONE ANALOGS

The advent of continuous-use GnRH analogs, particularly those in depot form, has facilitated hormonal preparation of the endometrium as these compounds produce a profound hypoestrogenic state and, subsequently, uniform atrophy of the endometrium. However, because they are agonists, there is usually a flare-up phase of 2–3 weeks before the desensitization phase, with a drop in gonadotropins. Although administration during the late luteal phase somewhat blunts the agonistic phase, the initial flare-up still occurs in most patients. When using depot forms such as depot Lupron 3.75 mg intramuscularly, endometrial ablation can be performed a month later. However, a significant number of patients will not achieve complete atrophy of the endometrium within this time owing to the variability of the flare-up phase which

may result in only 1–2 weeks of desensitization, which may not be sufficient for endometrial atrophy. Approximately 25–30% of patients may still have thickened endometrium following desensitization. For this reason, it is useful to give a second injection 4 weeks after the first to ensure complete and sufficient desensitization, and which may produce an atrophic endometrium in more than 95% of these patients (Figure 10.3).

Although most patients require a 3.75 mg intramuscular injection, some patients with marked obesity may benefit more from a 7.5-mg dose. Endometrial ablation is then scheduled to take place 2–3 weeks following the second injection.

Hormonal preparation of the endometrium is also useful in patients with submucous leiomyomas before they undergo resectoscopic or hysteroscopic myomectomy. The endometrium becomes thinner, permitting better visualization during myomectomy. Should patients bleed excessively, which is usually the case with these types of myomas, the procedure can be performed after the bleeding is controlled. This is particularly useful if the patient is anemic as it re-establishes normal levels of hemoglobin and permits, if necessary, storage of autologous blood. The use of GnRH analogs, which is now the preferred method for preparing these patients for surgery, provides additional benefits to facilitate myomectomy: decreased vascularization due to a reduced blood flow; some reduction in the size of the leiomyoma, which makes the procedure easier to perform; and a more predictable cessation of abnormal bleeding. In general, depot Lupron at 3.75 mg intramuscularly is administered in three doses as monthly injections. The decision whether to use

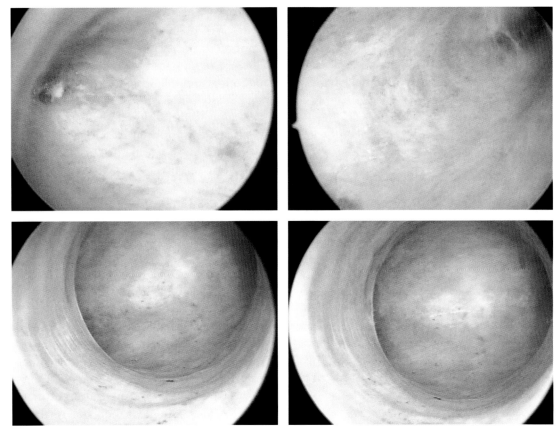

Figure 10.3 Hysteroscopic views of atrophic endometrium

these hormonal adjuncts or not is based on the individual patient, taking into account the bleeding, hemoglobin levels and size and type of leiomyoma, as those with an intramural component almost always require this type of preparation.

Other hysteroscopic therapeutic procedures that require good visualization of the uterine cavity, an absence of debris and a thin endometrium include division of uterine septa and tubal cannulation. In these cases, if the procedures are performed in the immediate postmenstrual period, hormonal preparation is usually not necessary. Those patients who bleed abnormally because of oligo-ovulation may benefit

from hormonal preparation of the endometrium (Table 10.1).

OTHER ADJUNCTS TO HYSTEROSCOPIC SURGERY

Prophylactic antibiotics

Prophylactic antibiotics are used routinely in the treatment of uterine septa. They are usually administered by intravenous injection during the operation with 3–4 days of oral maintenance treatment. Patients treated for intrauterine adhesions are also given prophylactic antibiotics preoperatively and

Table 10.1 Side-effects of preoperative medical treatments

GnRH agonists	Danazol	Progestogens
Hot flushes (90%)	Hot flushes (70%)	Fluid retention
Vaginal dryness	Fluid retention	Breast tenderness
Headaches	Mood swings	Weight gain
Breakthrough bleeding	Emotional instability	Persistent bleeding
Mood swings	Depression	Depression
Depression	Weight gain	Pseudodecidual reaction of endometrium
Decreased bone density,	Liver damage	
if prolonged	Loss of libido	
	Acne/seborrhea	

GnRH, gonadotropin-releasing hormone

for 3–4 days postoperatively as maintenance treatment if an intrauterine splint is not used. When intrauterine splints are used, the therapy is continued for 7 days orally, when the splint is removed.

Tubal cannulation may also require prophylactic antibiotics intraoperatively. The regimens vary, but the most commonly used antibiotics are the cephalosporins such as cephazolin or similar, 1 g intravenously 'piggyback' during the operation, followed by 500 mg of cephalexin orally four times a day. Alternatively, doxycycline 100 mg intravenously is used during the operation, piggybacked, followed by 100 mg twice daily orally for 4 days.

While the use of prophylactic antibiotics after removal of a uterine septum may not be uniformly accepted, because these patients are in a special category, such as infertility patients, extra care is taken to prevent the possibility of tubal infection.

Similarly, tubal cannulation requires manipulation of the tubal epithelium and may predispose the patient to infection, therefore, although on an empirical basis, the use of prophylactic antibiotics seems to be a reasonable approach.

Estrogen and progestogen treatment

Estrogen in the form of conjugated estrogens (Premarin®) is given in doses of 2.5 mg twice daily for 30 days after the division of uterine septa, followed by medroxyprogesterone acetate 10 mg/day orally during the last 7 days of the cycle to ensure withdrawal bleeding. Patients with moderate-to-severe intrauterine adhesions are also prescribed this estrogen regimen for 30–40 days. Although there is no evidence that these regimens are better than no treatment, on an empirical basis and by ultrasound measurements, they appear to expedite endometrial growth.

Hormonal preparations

For endometrial ablation, the following regimens are useful: danazol 800 mg/day in four doses for 6 weeks; depot Lupron 3.75 mg intramuscularly in two doses 1 month apart, except for patients who weigh more than 250 pounds (114 kg), in which case the dose is increased to 7.5 mg intramuscularly.

Myomas are also treated, if bleeding is excessive and continuous, the patient is anemic or the myoma is > 3 cm, with depot Lupron 3.75 mg intramuscularly (in three doses) 1 month apart. In anemic patients, the treatment may be continued until the hemoglobin and hematocrit levels are normalized.

Hysterosalpingogram

Hysterosalpingography or fluid-enhanced sonography is performed, if the patient desires pregnancy, 3 months after myomectomy to ensure that the symmetry of the uterine cavity is re-established. Following removal of intrauterine adhesions, hysterosalpingography can be performed after the hormonal treatment, particularly in moderate-to-severe cases, to ascertain normalcy of the uterine cavity and tubal patency. After division of a uterine septum and once hormonal treatment has been completed, a hysterosalpingogram should be obtained following menstruation to assess the symmetry of the uterine cavity. After tubal cannulation, a hysterosalpingogram is mandatory if pregnancy does not occur within 1 year.

Ultrasonography and fluid-enhanced sonography

Vaginal sonography is used preoperatively when leiomyomas are present, and postoperatively if the leiomyoma is partially intramural and not totally resected. Vaginal sonography should be performed to assess the status of the remaining partially treated leiomyoma 3–6 months following the procedure, or earlier if the patient becomes symptomatic. Fluid-enhanced sonography may also be carried out if the information obtained by vaginal sonography alone remains inadequate.

As a preoperative evaluation to submucous myomectomy, fluid-enhanced sonography becomes most useful to evaluate the degree of myoma penetration in the uterine wall, therefore outlining its size, shape and closeness to the serosal surface to evaluate feasibility and predict complete removal of the myoma (Figure 10.4).

Figure 10.4 Schematic representations of various types (0–II) of submucous myomas according to uterine wall penetration

SELECTED BIBLIOGRAPHY

Brooks PG, Serden SP, Davos I. Hormonal inhibition of the endometrium for resectoscopic endometrial ablation. *Am J Obstet Gynecol* 1991;164:1601

Droegemueller N, Herbst AL, Mishell DR, Stenchever MA. Abnormal uterine bleeding. In

Comprehensive Gynecology. St Louis: CV Mosby, 1987:953–64

Goldrath MH. Use of danazol in hysteroscopic surgery for menorrhagia. *J Reprod Med* 1990;35:91

Ke RW, Taylor PJ. Endometrial ablation to control excessive uterine bleeding. *Hum Reprod* 1991;6:574

Perino A, Chianchiano N, Petronio M, *et al*. Role of leuprolide acetate depot in hysteroscopic surgery: a controlled study. *Fertil Steril* 1993;59:507

Rich AD, Manyonda IT, Patel R, Amias AG. A comparison of the efficacy of danazol, norethisterone, cyproterone acetate and medroxyprogesterone acetate in endometrial thinning prior to ablation: a pilot study. *Gynaecol Endosc* 1995;4:59

Valle RF. Endometrial ablation for dysfunctional uterine bleeding: role of Gn-RH agonists. *Int J Gynecol Obstet* 1993;41:3

Valle RF. Assessing new treatments for dysfunctional uterine bleeding. *Contemp Obstet Gynecol* 1994;4:43

11

Video hysteroscopy and documentation

Diagnostic and therapeutic hysteroscopic procedures should be documented with diagrams, particularly in those cases that require operative intervention. It is important to outline and depict the findings and treatment in the diagram, particularly for those procedures that require follow-up and which may require additional procedures in the future. Simple drawings are useful as a complement to the operative report (Figure 11.1).

STILL PICTURES

While still pictures were used more extensively in the 1970s and 1980s as part of the documentation, with the advent of video, this valuable means of documentation has become somewhat neglected. Nevertheless, still photographs remain the best and simplest method of documenting important findings and important steps in an operative procedure. In addition, pictures in the

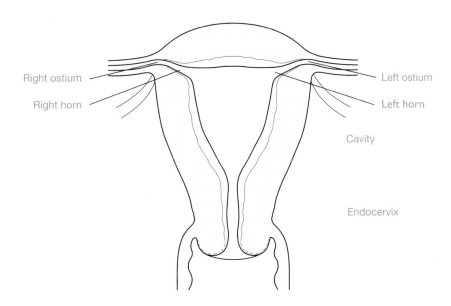

Figure 11.1 Sample report for documenting hysteroscopic examination findings

form of 35-mm transparencies are useful for educational purposes.

Digital photography, now a reality, has facilitated picture taking while the procedure is being performed, without the need for interruption and also concomitantly with videotaping.

VIDEO SYSTEMS

Video has become an integral part of endoscopy particularly because of its improved resolution and versatility. Small video cameras are easily adapted for attachment to the ocular parts of the hysteroscope or resectoscope, and operations can be performed under video monitoring. Video hysteroscopy was difficult before the new high-sensitivity cameras were introduced, particularly because of the need to provide powerful light sources to enable photography of the hysteroscopic procedures. At present, most cameras can be used through small endoscopes during diagnostic and operative procedures. Special cameras that are highly light-sensitive have been introduced specifically for this purpose (Figure 11.2). During operative procedures with a hysteroscope, the wide-angle view and high resolution of such a camera facilitates the performance of the procedure and confers greater accuracy when treating specific conditions. Similarly, when the resectoscope is used, the video camera permits a clearer view of the field and tissues, which is particularly important when dissecting, cutting or removing lesions (Figure 11.3). Video has also made it easier to assess different tissues, thereby rendering electrosurgery safer. In addition, the surgeon is able to operate in a comfortable position that does not require major effort, as is the case when the opera-

Figure 11.2 Highly light-sensitive camera specially designed for endoscopic procedures (Storz)

Figure 11.3 A three-chip video camera for endoscopy (Stryker)

tor must keep his eye to the hysteroscopic ocular during operations with endoscopes. Finally, the procedure is shared with the operating team, thus increasing interest, and enhancing their participation and help (Figure 11.4).

The new video printers and digital photographic units have greatly facilitated the production of video prints and slides with excellent color reproduction. Thus, there is no longer the necessity to interrupt both the videorecording of the operation and the operation itself to take a still photograph. Digital photography units can provide this

Figure 11.4 Video screen for viewing of endoscopic procedures (Stryker)

should be connected to the hysteroscope and/or resectoscope, the colors made uniform and the focusing completed. Moisture should be prevented from entering the ocular and camera lenses. If this occurs, the lenses should be cleaned with a soft dry cloth. The colors and brightness of the camera should be adapted as necessary, using conventional or standard light-sensitive cameras or a special camera with even greater sensitivity to light. The light source can be increased or decreased, according to requirements. Similarly, the zooming should be adapted according to the need.

Additionally, the introduction of CD-ROM to replace video cassettes has also enhanced the storing of important information that can be easily edited and reproduced for demonstration and teaching purposes.

type of documentation instantaneously; either the operator or an assistant can activate the unit at will whenever a photograph is required. This type of technology has become standard in most operating suites equipped with endoscopic systems.

PRACTICAL POINTS FOR VIDEO

It is important to prepare for videotaping before the procedure begins. The machine should be checked, a clean tape inserted and the machine activated. Should a video print function be available, the pedal to obtain such pictures should be placed close to the operator. Before introduction of the hysterscope into the patient, the camera

SELECTED BIBLIOGRAPHY

Acland RD. Photomicrography through the operating microscope. *Plast Reconstruct Surg* 1977;60:730

Brooks PG. Video endoscopy cameras and printers to assist surgeons. *Contemp OB/GYN Technol* 1989;43–7

Kent PR, Malinak R. Intraoperative photography. A sterile system. *Obstet Gynecol* 1978;52:365

Marlow J. Endoscopic photography. In Baggish MS, ed. *Gynecologic Endoscopy and Instrumentation. Clinical Obstetrics and Gynecology*. Hagerstown, MD: Harper & Row, 1983:359–65

Marlow JL. Hysteroscopic photography. In Baggish MS, Barbot J, Valle RF, eds. *Diagnostic and Operative Hysteroscopy. A Text and Atlas*. Chicago: Year Book Medical Publishers, 1989:215–22

12

Learning hysteroscopy and resectoscopy for credentialing

The learning process for any surgical procedure should begin with recognition of the normal anatomy and its abnormal variations. Therefore, diagnostic hysteroscopy should always be the first step in the learning curve.

There are several methods available today for learning diagnostic hysteroscopy. Inanimate models are most useful for testing the instruments and their direction of view – specifically, foreoblique vision – and the movements necessary for a general inspection. After inanimate models, the transition to animal models is easier; different distending media can be used and the mechanisms involved in working the various systems explored. Cow uteri and pig bladders are easily obtainable and can be mounted on small platforms; extirpated uteri after hysterectomy can also be used as models for learning the fundamentals of this type of endoscopy (Figure 12.1).

Once the instrumentation, different distending media and techniques have become familiar, the physician can perform the procedures in live patients in the operating room. It is useful to begin with a patient who is under general anesthesia, as this permits the use of the instruments without undue hesitation, thereby allowing more time for examination and dealing with any problems that may arise with the instrumentation; the operator is also free of any

worry of being observed by the patient. In general, patients who require curettage for evaluation of abnormal bleeding are excellent candidates. Before attempting the clinical application of these procedures, hysteroscopy should be performed in patients who have no pathology such as those who require tubal sterilization, or in patients prior to a vaginal hysterectomy.

The use of hysteroscopy therapeutically should only be attempted after having mastered the diagnostic techniques, as the therapeutic procedures require greater experience with the instruments. Inanimate models may be useful, such as plastic uterine models with pathological lesions that can be dissected and removed. Green peppers or melons can be used to simulate the uterus (Figure 12.2); different structures and multiple seeds can be grasped with grasping flexible or rigid forceps. Bands of tissue can be cut to simulate division of a septum or an adhesion. Cardboard boxes can be constructed into different obstacles that will serve as lesions to be removed or divided. The physician can then move on to animal models, for example cow uteri or pig bladders containing simulated pathological lesions, such as tissue sutured to the walls to simulate polyps or myomas, sutures in the midline to simulate a septum or sutures from wall to wall at different places to simulate adhesions. These exercises help to acquire dexterity in the

Figure 12.1 Different exercises for practicing procedures using extirpated uteri and simulated lesions

Figure 12.2 Model boxes devised for training use various materials to simulate lesions and anatomical structures

manipulation of semirigid or flexible instruments through the hysteroscopic operating channel. Furthermore, while operating, the direction of view can be changed from one place to another and the physician can observe the changes that occur within the simulated cavity and correlate them later to observations during an actual operation.

The use of the resectoscope also requires special instruction. The instrument should be well known in all its components, and assembled and disassembled to gain an understanding of how the various parts fit together in the system. The most often performed procedures with a resectoscope can be attempted on surfaces such as a raw potato to simulate myomas that can be resected with a loop while embedded in a non-electrolyte-containing fluid. Before the resectoscope is activated, special grounding of all these substances is necessary. Liver or other similar tissues can also be coagulated and resected under simulated circumstances. The transition is then made to extirpated pig bladders or cow uteri with different lesions attached, representing various pathological conditions to be resected and/or coagulated. The roller-ball/bar electrodes can be used to simulate endometrial ablation by coagulation in these specimens to demonstrate how these instruments are activated and rolled, and what their effect on tissues is.

Physicians who want to learn how to use fiberoptic lasers should use the operative hysteroscope with activated lasers on specimens simulating the human uterus. A bare fiber and both the contact or dragging technique and the non-contact blanching technique for coagulation should be used to learn their different effects on tissue. The same precautions (special goggles or filters) as those taken in the operating suite should be exercised when these lasers are used and activated to protect the eyes from retinal injury.

ANESTHESIA

At the beginning of the learning curve, most procedures, whether diagnostic or therapeutic, but particularly the latter, should be performed under general anesthesia. Once experience and confidence are acquired, diagnostic procedures can be attempted under local anesthesia. This is important not only to avoid frustration but, if the procedure does not go as planned, to prevent undue concern by the patient. Regional anesthesia is appropriate for most hysteroscopic and/or resectoscopic procedures unless laparoscopy is planned. Nevertheless, the patient's wishes should be respected as many will only accept general anesthesia. If cervical dilatation is required while using local anesthesia and the dilatation is difficult or the patient becomes uncomfortable, it is preferable to abort the procedure and change the anesthetic to make the patient comfortable. If local anesthesia fails to produce its effect and the operator persists in attempting to complete the cervical dilatation, the result may be more anxiety and a painful experience for the patient. Therefore, these patients require other anesthetics at different settings.

PRECEPTORSHIPS

Although diagnostic and operative hysteroscopy can be learned by reading, observing and reviewing photographs and videos, the availability of a preceptor is important. A preceptor can encourage progress, correct mistakes, expedite the learning curve and guide the practitioner in performing the procedure more safely. Preceptorships are most useful when operative procedures are to be learned, whether with a hysteroscope or resectoscope. A preceptor can help not only in the performance of a procedure itself, but also in setting the system up to be particularly effective for learning the procedure and in helping the assisting team, especially the nurses, to establish a standard arrangement for the instruments and any additional requirements, such as delivery of the distending media, placement of the video system and monitoring of electrical or laser energies. In addition, the preceptor can attest to the ability of the practitioner to perform specific procedures safely once the preceptorship is completed.

It is important, having learned the hysteroscopic/resectoscopic procedures, to maintain proficiency, as with any other surgical procedure.

Virtual reality, an advanced human–computer interaction where individuals can visualize, manipulate and interact with computers on a complex level, is now beginning to be used in hysteroscopy training. While its use is not widespread as yet, it certainly offers an excellent method of acquiring dexterity and proficiency in the treatment of various intrauterine conditions in an unhurried and non-threatening environment. This method offers great promise in the training of any endoscopic procedure to acquire necessary hand–eye co-ordination and dexterity.

ACCREDITATION AND CREDENTIALING

Because of the need to ensure safety and efficacy in carrying out new procedures, hospitals are beginning to credential physicians in these procedures necessitating the fulfillment of several requirements for the learning and acquisition of new skills. Accreditation only certifies that these requirements have been fulfilled. Accreditation councils cannot ensure credentialing, which is the responsibility of each institution that is to grant privileges to physicians to perform these or other surgical procedures.

Establishing credentials for hysteroscopy: requirements

(1) Privileges in gynecological surgery;

(2) Didactic course;

(3) Practical workshop (laboratory setting);

(4) Tutorial by qualified hysteroscopist;

(5) Supervision of first cases, particularly operative cases;

(6) Advanced procedures require preceptorship;

(7) Laser and resectoscope (special requirements);

(8) Experimental techniques: approved informed consent and protocol by Institutional Review Board.

The above monitoring methods will also ensure that those physicians who want to perform new procedures that they have not yet performed should undergo initial supervision until competency has been demonstrated.

Most credentialing institutions in the USA have adopted or modified the guidelines for obtaining privileges in gynecological operative endoscopy proposed by the Society of Reproductive Surgeons and the American Society of Reproductive Medicine (ASRM), formerly known as the American Fertility Society, in 1994.

We have adopted three levels of competency for hysteroscopy.

Level I: diagnostic hysteroscopy (elemental).

Level II: minor operative procedures (require some training):

(1) Targeted biopsies;
(1) Polypectomy (pedunculated, < 3 cm);
(1) Myomectomy (pedunculated, < 2 cm);
(1) Endometrial ablation by coagulation (roller-ball);
(1) Removal of misplaced IUDs;
(1) Lysis of central, focal adhesions;
(1) Division of partial, thin septa;
(1) Sterilization by ESSURE system.

Level III: More difficult operative procedures (require additional training and experience):

(1) Polypectomy (> 3 cm or sessile);
(1) Myomectomy (> 2 cm or with intramural component);
(1) Endometrial ablation by electrosurgical resection or laser photovaporization;
(1) Tubal cannulation for cornual obstruction;
(1) Division of complete or broad septa;
(1) Extensive adhesions with complete cavity occlusion.

While residency programs now offer training in endoscopy, laparoscopy and hysteroscopy, the training *per se* has not been formalized uniformly; therefore, it still depends on observation and assisting in various procedures, and it is left up to the instructor to decide which ones and when the resident can perform them under supervision. However, because of the increased variety and number of surgical cases, residency programs are in an enviable position to offer residents experience with a variety of pathological conditions that will help them better to learn and understand hysteroscopic surgery.

All therapeutic hysteroscopic procedures require knowledge of diagnostic hysteroscopy. All practitioners must show evidence of having: attended a formal course on indications, contraindications and possible complications; attended a laboratory workshop designed to teach how to perform these procedures; knowledge of physics and the basic principles of electrosurgery as well as laser energies; appropriate credentialing in the performance of minor and major gynecological procedures.

SELECTED BIBLIOGRAPHY

American College of Gynecologists and Obstetricians. *Credentialing Guidelines for New Operative Procedures*, ACGO Committee Opinion, No. 142. Washington, DC: ACGO, 1994

American College of Surgeons. Statement of emerging surgical technologies and the evaluation of credentials. *Am Coll Surg Bull* 1994;79:40

Barak G. The learning curve [Editorial]. *J Am Med Assoc* 1993;270:1280

Cass OW, Freeman ML, Peine CJ, *et al.* Objective evaluation of endoscopy skills during training. *Ann Intern Med* 1993;118:40

Gimpelson RJ, Schomburg ME, Bagby ML. An animal model for learning Nd : YAG laser ablation of the endometrium. *J Reprod Med* 1989;39:461

Hatlie MJ. Climbing 'the learning curve'. New technologies, emerging obligations. *J Am Med Assoc* 1989;270:1364

Keye WR. Hitting a moving target: credentialing the endoscopic surgeon. *Fertil Steril* 1994; 62:1115

Lefebvre Y, Cote J, Lefebvre L. Teaching surgical hysteroscopy by virtual simulation. In Phillips JM, Hunt RB, Loffer FD, eds. *Hysteroscopy Update*. Santa Fe Springs, CA: The American Association of Gynecological Laparoscopy, 1997;177–8

Sanmarco MJ, Youngblood JP. A resident teaching program in operative endoscopy. *Obstet Gynecol* 1993;81:463

Siegler AM. Learning and teaching hysteroscopic tubal sterilization. In Sciarra JJ, Butler JC, Speidel JJ, eds. *Hysteroscopic Sterilization*. New York: Intercontinental Medical Book Corporation, 1974:113–43

Society for Reproductive Surgeons and The American Fertility Society. Guidelines for attaining privileges in gynecologic operative endos-copy. *Fertil Steril* 1994;62:1118

Tulandi T. Canadian guidelines for training in operative endoscopy [Letter to the Editor]. *Gynaecol Endosc* 1995;4:69

Valle RF. Training and Accreditation: USA. Training, proctoring and credentialing. In Van Herendael BJ, Valle RF, Bettocchi S, eds. *Ambulatory Hysteroscopy: Diagnostic and Operative*. London: Bladon Medical Publishing, 2004:184–7

Wolfe WM, Levine RL, Sanfilippo JS, Eggler S. A teaching model for endoscopic surgery: hysteroscopy and pelviscopy surgery. *Fertil Steril* 1988;50:662

13

Hysterosalpingography and laparoscopy in infertility

Alvin M. Siegler

It has been estimated that approximately 300 000 diagnostic hysterosalpingograms (HSGs) are done in the United States annually and many examinations are performed with spot films without fluoroscopy[1]. In a recent review of hospitals in Liverpool, England, Hugh reported that approximately 100 HSGs were done each year in the hospitals surveyed[2]. One-third of hysterosalpingograms are administered only by radiologists, another third by gynecologists alone, and in the rest of the patients both physicians are involved.

Hysterosalpingography (HSG) is an important screening procedure during an investigation of infertility, even though the procedure cannot detect endometriosis or significant pelvic adhesions (Table 13.1).

TECHNIQUE

HSG is performed in the preovulatory phase as an outpatient procedure. Less than 20% of women require sedation or antispasmodic agents. Patients with a history of pelvic inflammatory disease should be given antibacterial prophylaxis. Water-soluble contrast material is injected through either a metal cannula or a Foley catheter balloon. The study usually requires 4–5 spot films to be taken under

fluoroscopic image intensification using 6–8 ml of contrast material, the amount depending on the size of the uterine cavity (Figure 13.1)[3].

Proximal tubal obstruction is suspected if the cornua are pointed rather than rounded, with absence of tubal filling after contrast material has been injected. Tubal filling with spill and spread of the contrast material on the drainage film indicates tubal patency, although the proximal segment always should be examined for tubal polyps or diverticula.

Technical variations include the use of 70- and 105-mm radiographs, technetium-99 HSG as an alternative to contrast HSG[4] cinefluoroscopy, low-dose scanning-beam digital HSG, and radionuclide studies to assess tubal patency[5]. An attempt to correlate tubal perfusion pressures and opacification by standardizing the injection volume per time interval has been described[6].

Errors in technique and interpretation of HSGs are frequently causes for discrepancies when the results are compared with the findings at laparoscopy. The most common reason for failure to see the uterine cavity is inadequate traction on the cervix or obstruction of the view of the lower uterine segment because of either the catheter bulb (Figure 13.2) or an opaque speculum[7]. Failure to opacify tubes can be caused by

Table 13.1 Hysterosalpingography as a screen for intrauterine and tubal causes of infertility

Uterine cavity
Normal triangular shape
Congenital uterine anomalies
Intrauterine adhesions
Submucous tumors
    polyps/myomas

Fallopian tubes
Diagnostically
    normal fill-and-spill
    intramural polyps
    salpingitis isthmica nodosa
    endometriosis/tuberculosis
    hydrosalpinx
    operability
    prognosis for fertility
Therapeutically
    normal Fallopian tubes
    use of OBCM for fertility enhancement
    proximal tubal obstruction
    selective salpingography and cannulation

Accuracy
Excellent for uterine cavity disease screening
Screening for Fallopian tube disease
    normal
    suspicious
    abnormal
Poor for endometriosis/periadnexal disease screening

Common errors
Failure to opacify entire uterine cavity
    axial view
    failed cervical traction
    balloon-catheter technique
    opaque vaginal speculum
Failure to evaluate Fallopian tubes properly
    endpoints fill/spill or
    increased abdominal pain/intravasation
    no drainage film
    mucosal pattern obscured

OBCM, oil-based contrast medium

the use of inadequate amounts of contrast material. The endpoint of stopping the injection should be either an increase in lower abdominal pain or evidence of vascular intravasation. Failure to obtain a drainage film will prevent adequate evaluation of the filled tube and miss the diagnosis of fimbrial phimosis. The delayed film helps to differentiate distal tubal obstruction from tubal patency.

Figure 13.1 This enlarged uterine cavity (d) was caused by a submucous myoma. Fractional instillation of contrast material (a)–(c) outlines the cavity and reveals the defect

Figure 13.2 A common technical error in hysterosalpingography is caused by failure to exert sufficient traction on the cervical tenaculum (a). The balloon catheter is inserted too far into the uterine cavity (b)

Tubes are considered normal if bilateral tubal fill-and-spill is seen with normal rugae markings and without localization on the drainage film (Figure 13.3). The isthmic segment should show a thin linear opacification. An abnormal salpingogram is defined by the presence of distal tubal occlusion with or without a hydrosalpinx. A salpingogram is considered suspicious or equivocal when there is partial tubal filling, proximal tubal obstruction is seen or different sites of occlusion are found in each tube.

A HSG that is performed adequately and carefully interpreted remains an excellent screening test for uterine and tubal abnormalities because of its ability to outline the lumina of the Fallopian tubes and uterine cavity. The examination should be able to detect congenital uterine abnormalities, intrauterine adhesions and submucous

Figure 13.3 Normal appearances of the Fallopian tube on hysterosalpingography include clear rugal markings (arrows)

tumors such as polyps or myomas (Figures 13.4 and 13.5).

CONTRAST MATERIAL

What is the therapeutic effect of the HSG? Pregnancy rates following the use of oil-based contrast material (OBCM) and water-based contrast materials (WBCM) have been confounded by a number of variables. In an effort to compare the therapeutic effects of OBCM and WBCM, 29 patients who had a normal pelvic anatomy at laparoscopy were randomized to receive either OBCM ($n = 15$) or WBCM ($n = 014$). A significant difference in pregnancy rates was noted: 40% in those receiving OBCM and 14% in the WBCM group. These observations were confirmed in another study which showed significantly more term pregnancies with the use of an ethiodized poppyseed oil for HSG than with the use of

three water-soluble contrast media groups[8,9]. A potential mechanism for fertility enhancement was suggested by a study which showed the ability of contrast material and/or indigo–carmine dye to inhibit lymphocytic proliferation and phagocytosis by macrophages in the peritoneal fluid[10].

CATHETERIZATION

Although the debate about the selection of the best contrast material is ongoing, one of the most significant additions to HSG has been the introduction of interventional and imaging techniques that offer new therapeutic possibilities[11–14]. The diagnosis of proximal tubal obstruction made by HSG and confirmed by laparoscopy is not followed invariably by tubocornual anastomosis because transcervical selective salpingography (TSS) is available as the contemporary approach to non-opacification of the Fallopian tube. Fluoroscopically guided coaxial catheterization and canalization has resulted in tubal patency in so many patients that the procedure has become a prerequisite before attempting microsurgical anastomosis. The data suggest that these procedures are the best first choice for the most definitive diagnosis or treatment. Such an approach requires renewed co-operation between the gynecologist and radiologist, leading to the suggestion by Gleicher and colleagues[15] to form a Gynecoradiology Special Interest Group as a section within the American Society of Reproductive Medicine.

After a HSG has shown either unilateral or bilateral proximal tubal obstruction, TSS is carried out. The transcervical approach to the intramural and isthmic tubal segments is less invasive than tubo-

Figure 13.4 (a) Multiple intrauterine filling defects resulted from endometrial polyps. (b) Severe intrauterine distortion was caused by advanced intrauterine adhesions. (c) Myometrial intravasation was caused by adenomyosis. (d) The effects of diethylstilbestrol *in utero* produced a tubal bulge (open arrow) and an intrauterine defect (solid arrow) in this patient

cornual anastomosis. It is capable of restoring patency to apparent proximal tubal obstruction seen on the HSG that had been caused by spasm, debris and filmy adhesions[16]. Capitanio and co-workers[17] used the technique in 108 women who had proximal tubal obstruction (59 unilateral, 49 bilateral) on HSG. Under fluoroscopy, after paracervical block, a repeat HSG was performed. When proximal tubal obstruction was confirmed, a 4.5-Fr (1.5 mm) catheter was inserted through an 8-Fr (2.7 mm) introducer and wedged into the tubal ostium, then advanced to the

Figure 13.5 Fallopian tube shows bipolar disease with salpingitis isthmica nodosa (sin) and hydro-salpinx (H)

tubal isthmus. If an obstruction was not met, the coaxial guidewire was passed through the catheter. The catheter was advanced over the guidewire, the guidewire removed and 2–3 ml of contrast material injected to verify canalization. The opposite tube was treated with the same procedure. A conventional HSG was carried out at the end of the TSS procedure. In 108 women, 155 tubes were catheterized whereas nine could not be catheterized. Of the 146 successfully treated tubes, 110 became patent, 21 showed distal occlusion, ten showed partial distal occlusion and the remaining five showed midtubal obstruction; there were two instances of tubal perforation. Of the 46 women who had 'successful' tubal canalization, only four achieved term pregnancies and none had tubal pregnancies.

In most series, the proximally obstructed tube can be catheterized and tubal patency demonstrated in more than 80% of patients[18–22]. Thus, tubocornual anastomosis has become a relatively infrequent operation and the standard of care dictates that, in women undergoing HSG or at

laparoscopy, TSS is essential prior to tubal microsurgery or *in vitro* (IVF). In an attempt to standardize HSG and TSS, Gleicher and colleagues[6] measured tubal perfusion pressures during TSS and correlated them with tubal opacification. The authors noted a wide range of pressures (429 ± 376 mmHg), which were significantly lower than those seen in abnormal-looking tubes (957 ± 445 mmHg). These results suggest that the concomitant performance of perfusion pressure studies during TSS enhances its capability to detect abnormalities in the Fallopian tubes.

Another variation of non-operative tubal patency studies was reported by Tufekci and co-workers[23], who performed transvaginal sonosalpingography (TVSOS) using 10–20 ml of isotonic saline injected into the uterine cavity through a catheter. In 39 women, TVSOS accurately showed patency in 29 patients and bilateral non-patency in three. When compared with laparoscopy in ten women, the results were confirmed partially. Intratubal flow was followed for 5 s through each tube and fimbrial turbulence or cul-de-sac fluid accumulation was considered evidence of patency of at least one tube. TVSOS indicated patency or non-patency of one or both tubes in 37 of 38 patients. The results were confirmed by subsequent chromotubation at laparoscopy with 1% methylene blue. The advantages over HSG claimed by the authors were its greater potential safety, greater convenience and lower cost, its lack of potential interaction with contrast media, and the fact that it is a simple post-operative test following tubal anastomosis.

Both HSG and laparoscopy have some predictability as regards pregnancy outcome following microsurgical neosalpingostomy[24–26]. On HSG, the mucosal pattern as

Table 13.2   Predictive value of hysterosalpingography and laparoscopy in hydrosalpinx

Hysterosalpingogram
Mucosal pattern
Diameter of hydrosalpinx
Expansibility of ampulla

Laparoscopy
Extent and type of periadnexal adhesions
Thickness of tubal wall
Diameter of hydrosalpinx

evidenced by the presence or absence of the dark line in the ampulla, and the diameter of the hydrosalpinx and its expansibility, are characteristics to be sought in evaluating the salpingogram. The most important feature is the radiological character of the mucosal pattern. During laparoscopy or laparotomy, the extent and nature of the adhesions, the thickness of the tubal wall and the diameter of the hydrosalpinx affect the postoperative prognosis for fertility (Table 13.2).

Opsahl and colleagues[27] conducted laparoscopy in 766 patients at 2–9 months after HSG and noted that a normal HSG was confirmed at laparoscopy in 326 of 327 patients, a 96.6% accuracy. In abnormal tubes, 89 of 93 HSGs were confirmed at laparoscopy. The largest differences between the findings of the two tests were in the 336 HSGs with equivocal findings. Moderate-to-severe non-pelvic disease can occur occasionally in women despite a normal HSG and, thus, laparoscopy should be done in such patients when other factors have been corrected and pregnancy has not occurred.

Salpingograms with equivocal findings should be confirmed by laparoscopy because the radiological results could be false-positive (proximal tubal obstruction caused by spasm or debris) or there may be

significant pelvic disease. Diagnostic laparoscopy can locate and stage endometriosis, classify the severity of periadnexal adhesions, examine the uterine serosal surface and evaluate the size, consistency and patency of the Fallopian tubes. The endoscopic examination can study more precisely the fimbriated ends of the Fallopian tubes. The distally obstructed tubes in certain instances are not amenable to operative repair and, in other situations, the prognosis for pregnancy postoperatively is so low that patients should be spared even a laparoscopy and entered directly into an IVF or adoption program.

Although many gynecologists use HSG as a screening procedure to establish tubal disease preoperatively, few studies have been carried out to assess its sensitivity and specificity following tubal microsurgery. Letterie and co-workers[28] correlated HSG and laparoscopy findings after tubal anastomosis in 11 patients and following distal salpingostomies in 14 patients. HSG was able to assess accurately the presence of tubal patency, but was limited in its ability to detect tubal adhesions. Thus, a screening HSG is indicated in the postoperative patient who has not achieved a pregnancy within 6 months. If recurrent tubal occlusion is noted, then IVF is advised but, if patency is seen, then another 6 months

Table 13.3 Features of laparoscopy

Diagnostic value
Detects endometriosis
Locates periadnexal adhesions
Examines uterus
    serosal surface only
Evaluates tubes
    serosal surface, consistency, delineation of fimbria
Therapeutic role
Endometriosis
Lyses periadnexal adhesions
Neosalpingostomy
Monitors hysteroscopic cannulation
Tubal anastomosis for reversal of tubal sterilization and myomectomy in selected instances

should elapse before a repeat laparoscopy is indicated to search for periadnexal adhesions.

HSG used preoperatively in planning a myomectomy can detect the contours of the uterine cavity and ascertain the patency of the Fallopian tubes[29]. Postoperatively, possible intrauterine adhesions or myometrial defects can be observed and the impact of the operation on the Fallopian tubes reassessed. Another possible use of HSG is in the early differential diagnosis of an intrauterine pregnancy from an intratubal abortion in patients who have declining or low levels of human chorionic gonadotropin (hCG). Of four patients in whom transvaginal sonography could not confirm pregnancy, three showed the characteristic finding of a tubal pregnancy on HSG. A normal-looking uterine cavity with the finding of a small saccular diverticulum arising from the tubal isthmus is apparently diagnostic. In contrast, a missed intrauterine abortion shows a characteristic abnormal uterine cavity[30]. In association with low positive hCG titers and an apparently normal uterine cavity, this radiological picture should suggest a strong suspicion that an early tubal pregnancy has occurred. HSG studies should be performed only after the hCG values have declined significantly. It is suggested that HSG be done in patients who have so-called biochemical pregnancy losses and a history of tubal disease or previous tubal surgery. The clinical implication for the patient who has radiologic evidence of a tubal pregnancy is that she is likely to have another tubal pregnancy.

SUMMARY

Hysterosalpingography remains an excellent screening examination to search for intrauterine and tubal causes of infertility. The findings can avoid the need for laparoscopy in some patients with advanced tubal abnormalities. In selected patients, HSG can be therapeutic, as suggested by the results of the use of oil-soluble media in patients with unexplained infertility and the use of interventional coaxial tubal catheterization for proximal tubal obstruction. Laparoscopy (Table 13.3) is both diagnostic and therapeutic, and has a wide range of applications requiring minimally invasive surgery. The use of these two procedures should be considered essential in the management of the infertile patient.

REFERENCES

1. Yoder IC, Hall DA. Hysterosalpingography in the 1990s. *Am J Radiol* 1991;157:675–83

2. Hugh AE. The role of hysterosalpingography in modern gynecological practice. *Br J Radiol* 1993;66:278–9

3. Hunt RB, Siegler AM. *Hysterosalpingography: Techniques and Interpretation.* Chicago: Year Book Medical, 1990

4. Angtuaco TL, Boyd CM, London SN, *et al.* Technetium-99 hysterosalpingography in infertility: an accurate alternative to contrast hysterosalpingography. *Radiographics* 1989; 9:115–28

5. Jacobson A, Uszler JM. A simplified technique for radionuclide hysterosalpingography. *J Assist Reprod Genet* 1993;10:4–10

6. Gleicher N, Parrilli M, Redding L, *et al.* Standardization of hysterosalpingography and selective salpingography: a valuable adjunct to simple opacification studies. *Fertil Steril* 1992;58:1136–41

7. Hofman GE, Scott RT, Rosenwaks Z. Common technical errors in hysterosalpingography. *Int J Fertil* 1992;37:41–3

8. Letterie GS, Rose GS. Pregnancy rates after the use of oil-based and water-based contrast media to evaluate tubal patency. *South Med J* 1990;83:1402–3

9. Rasmussen F, Lindequist S, Larsen C, *et al.* Therapeutic effect of hysterosalpingography: oil- versus water-soluble contrast media, a randomized prospective study. *Radiology* 1991;179:75–8

10. Goodman SB, Rein MS, Hill JA. Hysterosalpingography contrast media and chromopertubation dye inhibit peritoneal lymphocyte and macrophage function *in vitro*: a potential mechanism for fertility enhancement. *Fertil Steril* 1993;59:1022–7

11. Lisse K, Sydow P. Fallopian tube catheterization and recanalization under ultrasonic observation: a simplified technique to evaluate tubal patency and open proximally obstructed tubes. *Fertil Steril* 1991; 56:198–203

12. Martensson O, Nilsson B, Ekelund L, *et al.* Selective salpingography and fluoroscopic transcervical salpingoplasty for diagnosis and treatment of proximal tube occlusions. *Acta Obstet Gynecol Scand* 1993;72:458–64

13. Isaacson KB, Amendola M, Banner B, *et al.* Transcervical fallopian tube recanalization: a safe and effective therapy for patients with proximal tubal obstruction. *Int J Fertil* 1992;37:106–10

14. Thurmond AS, Rosch J. Nonsurgical fallopian tube recanalization for treatment of infertility. *Radiology* 1990;174:371–4

15. Gleicher N, Thurmond AS, Burry KA, *et al.* Gynecoradiology: a new approach to diagnosis and treatment of tubal disease. *Fertil Steril* 1992;58:885–7

16. Sulak PJ, Letterie GS, Coddington CC, *et al.* Histology of proximal tubal occlusion. *Fertil Steril* 1987;48:437–40

17. Capitanio GL, Ferraiolo A, Croce S, *et al.* Transcervical selective salpingography: a diagnostic and therapeutic approach to cases of proximal tubal obstruction. *Fertil Steril* 1991;55:1045–50

18. Confino E, Tur-Kaspa I, DeCherney A, *et al.* Transcervical balloon tuboplasty: a multicenter study. *J Am Med Assoc* 1990;264:2079–82

19. Burke P, Sabia A, Di Virgilio MR, *et al.* Indications for tubal recanalisation in diagnostic and interventional hysterosalpingography. *Radiol Med* 1993;85:657–61

20. Kumpe DA, Zwerdlinger SC, Rothbarth LJ, *et al.* Proximal fallopian tube occlusion: diagnosis and treatment with transcervical fallopian tube catheterization. *Radiology* 1990; 177:183–7

21. Lang EK, Dunaway HE Jr, Roniger WE. Selective osteal salpingography and transcer-

vical catheter dilatation in the diagnosis and treatment of fallopian tube obstruction. *Am J Radiol* 1990;154:735–8

22. Lederer KJ. Transcervical tubal cannulation and salpingoscopy in the treatment of tubal infertility. *Curr Opin Obstet Gynecol* 1993; 5:240–4

23. Tufekci EC, Girit S, Bayirli E, *et al*. Evaluation of tubal patency by transvaginal sonosalpingography. *Fertil Steril* 1992; 57:336–40

24. Henig I, Prough SG, Cheatwood M, *et al*. Hysterosalpingography, laparoscopy and hysteroscopy in infertility. A comparative study. *J Reprod Med* 1991;36:573–5

25. te Velde ER, Boer-Meisel ME, Meisner J, *et al*. The significance of preoperative hysterosalpingography and laparoscopy for predicting pregnancy outcome in patients with a bilateral hydrosalpinx. *Eur J Obstet Gynecol Reprod Biol* 1989;31:33–45

26. Schnack Peen UB, Pelle J, Bostofte E, *et al*. Hysterosalpingography, pre- and postoperative laparoscopy in operative treatment of infertility. *Acta Eur Fertil* 1989;20:355–8

27. Opsahl MS, Miller B, Klein TA. The predictive value of hysterosalpingography for tubal and peritoneal infertility factors. *Fertil Steril* 1993;60:444–8

28. Letterie GS, Haggerty MF, Fellows DW. Sensitivity of hysterosalpingography after tubal surgery. *Arch Gynecol Obstet* 1992; 251:175–80

29. Karasick S, Ehrlich S. The value of hysterosalpingography before reversal of sterilization procedures involving the fallopian tubes. *Am J Radiol* 1989;153:1247–50

30. Gleicher N, Parilli M, Pratt DE. Hysterosalpingography and selective salpingography in the differential diagnosis of chemical intrauterine versus tubal pregnancy. *Fertil Steril* 1993;57:553–8

14

Vaginal ultrasound, hysterosonography, three-dimensional imaging and Doppler for gynecological imaging

Leeber Cohen

During the early 1990s, it became increasingly common for gynecologists to perform office and emergency-room transvaginal ultrasound procedures. Although there is controversy surrounding training and credentialing, the need for a basic understanding of the instrumentation and principles of gynecological ultrasonography is clear. This has been best demonstrated by the rapid and accurate evaluation of suspect ectopic pregnancy in the emergency-room setting using transvaginal ultrasound (TVS)[1].

TVS, which is usually performed with an empty bladder, allows the clinician to image the uterus and adnexa to a high degree of resolution at the time of pelvic examination. This is particularly helpful in obese women and patients with abdominal guarding where pelvic examination is difficult. Common causes of menorrhagia, such as polyps and submucous leiomyomata, can be evaluated, and the risk for endometrial hyperplasia or endometrial cancer in women with postmenopausal bleeding determined by measuring the endometrial stripe. Suspect adnexal masses on bimanual examination can be visualized and the appropriate management determined.

Once comfortable with TVS imaging, many physicians are now performing their own sonohysterograms to identify space occupying lesions of the uterine cavity. Submucous leiomyomas can be measured and the degree of myometrial penetration determined. This chapter reviews transvaginal imaging as applied to gynecological imaging. The potential of three-dimensional (3-D) imaging and Doppler mapping of vasculature is also explored.

INSTRUMENTATION

The usual ultrasound machine for the gynecological office comes equipped with a variable frequency 3.5–5.0-MHz curvilinear transabdominal probe and a 5.0–7.5-MHz transvaginal probe. The initial set-up should be carried out by a qualified applications specialist sent by the manufacturer. The mechanical index should be adjusted to use the lowest power output needed for satisfactory images. Presettings for preprocessing, postprocessing, focus zones and filters should be set so that a minimum of adjustment is required by the practitioner.

Major advantages and disadvantages of the transabdominal and transvaginal probes compared with each other should be emphasized. The 3.5-MHz curvilinear probe is designed to give a wide-angle view (150°) of the pelvis; its lower frequency allows visualization of structures located up to 14 cm from the transducer. Masses that are large or located high in the pelvis should be evaluated by transabdominal ultrasound. The 7.5-MHz transvaginal probe yields a 90° view and can visualize structures close to the vaginal apex with a high degree of resolution. However, there is rapid attenuation of sound, and structures lying > 8 cm away are poorly seen. Not all cases require the use of both types of ultrasound, although, occasionally, both techniques may be necessary. Good clinical judgment and experience are certainly required.

The first session that a resident spends in the department should be devoted to familiarization with the equipment, and a review of the involved physics and procedures. The session should include the proper attachment and removal of transducers to avoid damage to the connecting pins. Proper cleansing of transducers and sterilization of vaginal probes must be emphasized. Approved agents and requirements will vary from one country to the next. A gel or lubricant interface is to be used both inside and outside the probe cover for proper transmission of sound. The physician should be familiar with the location of the on–off switch, overall-gain control, fine-gain controls (time-gain compensation (TGC) toggles) and magnification controls, and the measurement software. The patient's name should be placed at the beginning of the examination and all pictures well labeled.

Figure 14.1 Transabdominal longitudinal images. Standard orientation used in the USA (left): the front of the transducer is imaged on the left and the inferior aspect of the bladder is on the right. In the non-standard orientation (right), the image is rotated 180° by orientating the front of the transducer to the right side of the image

ORIENTATION

The most difficult concept to teach in gynecological ultrasound is orientation. Both the ultrasound probe and the image must be oriented to allow the practitioner to interpret the image correctly. Most ultrasound laboratories in the USA orientate the front of the transducer to the left side of the screen (Figure 14.1). Most machines designate this orientation by an arrow or symbol at the top of the screen. For transabdominal ultrasound, most ultrasound units in the USA image longitudinal midline pictures with the patient's bladder showing on the right side of the screen, accomplished by aiming the front of the transducer, indicated on the transducer by a longitudinal groove or label, towards the patient's head. If the bladder does not appear on the right side of the screen (see Figure 14.1), the left–right inverse switch needs to be changed. For transverse images (Figure 14.2), the front of the transducer is aimed to

Figure 14.2 Transabdominal transverse images. In the standard orientation used by most radiologists in the USA (left), the front of the transducer is imaged on the left side of the screen; the patient's right side is displayed on the left and the patient's left is on the right. In the nonstandard orientation (right), the image can be rotated 180° by reversing the orientation of the transducer (indicated by a little arrow at top of screen)

Figure 14.3 Many ultrasound laboratories orientate the front of the transducer to the left side of the screen so that the cervix and vagina are at the top of the image with the uterine fundus below. (Left) The uterus is antroverted (rotated towards the bladder); (right) the same image with the front of the transducer displayed on the right side of the screen.

the patient's right; the patient's left side will then appear on the right, and vice versa. The orientation of the probe and the image must be checked at the beginning of each scan and vigilance maintained to avoid accidentally changing it.

Multiple orientations have been suggested for TVS displays. However, most ultrasound centers scan with the front of the vaginal transducer displayed on the left side of the screen. Aiming the front of the transducer at the bladder will result in an image of the bladder on the left side of the screen, whereas the cervix or vagina are usually displayed at the superior aspect of the image and the uterine fundus inferiorly. Anteversion or retroversion can be determined by the relative position of the uterus to the bladder (Figure 14.3).

The physician performing a transvaginal scan needs to be aware of the increased anxiety produced by this scan in some women.

The length of the probe is potentially alarming, so the depth of insertion and manipulation of the probe should be explained to the patient prior to the examination. With patients who appear to be nervous or have difficulty in relaxing for the examination, it may be better to have them insert the vaginal probe themselves.

If possible, both a physician and a sonographer should be present during the examination, one to perform the transvaginal procedure, the other to adjust and record the images on the machine. One person alone may perform both functions, but this requires practice to avoid any awkwardness. Furthermore, the second person may also serve as a chaperon.

As already mentioned, the vaginal probe should be carefully cleaned prior to use. A probe cover is mandatory. Ultrasound jelly should be applied to the inside of the probe cover and adequate lubricant spread on the outer surfaces. The transducer should be gently introduced in a longitudinal direction. If the bladder has not been completely emptied, the patient should be asked to try again. Images of the cervix, lower uterine segment and fundus should be obtained in both longitudinal and transverse planes, and the adnexa identified. These are usually located between the uterus and the iliac vessels, which serve as a landmark. The adnexa and any masses should be measured in three dimensions. The cul-de-sac should be imaged and the presence of fluid or clot-like echoes noted and measured.

The depth of insertion, plane of the long axis and lateral position of the transducer all require adjustment to achieve proper images of these structures. This is most easily accomplished when the patient's feet are placed in stirrups, thereby allowing adequate abduction of the legs. If stirrups are not available, imaging an anteverted uterus may be difficult, although elevating the patient's hips with a pad or pillow should help.

TVS IN CLINICAL SITUATIONS

Early pregnancy loss and ectopic pregnancy

The evaluation of early pregnancy bleeding and suspected ectopic pregnancy has been greatly eased by the transvaginal probe. The orderly appearance of the gestational sac at 28–35 days, the yolk sac at 35–48 days and the fetal pole at 42–56 days has been demonstrated by Warren and colleagues[2] (Figures 14.4 and 14.5), using transvaginal ultrasound and β-human chorionic gonadotropin (hCG) titers as standardized by the First International Reference

Figure 14.4 Transvaginal picture of a 5 mm early intrauterine gestational sac (straight arrow) is identified adjacent to the endometrial cavity (curved arrows)

Figure 14.5 Transvaginal image showing a 5 mm yolk sac with an adjacent 3-mm fetal pole (straight arrow)

Preparation. Discriminatory β-hCG values using the 3rd International Standard are approximately 1500 IU/l for the gestational sac, 7000 IU/l for the yolk sac and 17 000 IU/l for the fetal pole with heartbeat[3]. As a number of different β-hCG assay kits using three different standard preparations are currently available, practitioners need to establish β-hCG discriminatory zones for each laboratory involved. Serial titers should not be performed at two different laboratories as the results may then be discrepant.

Two additional important precautions should be taken when interpreting β-hCG titers. Multiple gestation can result in elevated titers that do not correlate with the expected embryonic structures. Patients with complete or incomplete abortion may have titers elevated to above the discriminatory zone for visualizing a gestational sac. Unnecessary operative interventions may occur if the clinician does not consider all of the clinical presentation data, including patient history, and pelvic examination, laboratory and ultrasound findings.

A yolk sac or a 2–3 mm fetal pole is usually seen when the mean intrauterine gestational sac diameter is 10 mm. If the gestational sac has achieved this size and a yolk sac or fetal pole are not seen, then the TVS should be repeated within 1 week. If these structures are still not seen, a diagnosis of missed abortion can be made. A diagnosis of early pregnancy loss can also be made when the mean gestational sac diameter is greater than 20 mm and a fetal pole with cardiac activity is not seen[4]. The diagnosis of a missed abortion can also be made by TVS when a fetal pole ≥ 5 mm fails to exhibit cardiac activity[5].

In women with first-trimester bleeding, subchorionic bleeds are frequently identified on ultrasonography. Although the published literature is scanty, it is generally accepted that the larger the bleed, the greater the likelihood of eventual miscarriage (Figure 14.6).

Timor-Tritsch and colleagues[1] have noted that ectopic pregnancies can be properly diagnosed with TVS in the emergency-room setting with a high degree of certainty. In approximately 30% of cases, the ectopic gestational sac can be visualized

Figure 14.6 Transvaginal image showing a subchorionic bleed, identified by hypoechoic echoes, dissecting between the chorion and uterine wall (straight arrow)

Figure 14.7 Transvaginal image of a tubal pregnancy (3.4 × 3.0 cm) with fetal pole and yolk sac

(Figure 14.7). In the remainder, the absence of an intrauterine gestational sac and the presence of a complex adnexal mass or hemoperitoneum allow the diagnosis of ectopic pregnancy with a high degree of accuracy. Care must be taken not to confuse a cystic corpus luteum with an ectopic gestational sac (Figure 14.8).

It may be difficult to differentiate an early intrauterine gestational sac from a pseudogestational sac, which can be seen in

Figure 14.8 Transvaginal image displaying a cystic corpus luteum and early intrauterine gestational sac. The corpus luteum is easily confused with an ectopic gestation

Figure 14.9 Transvaginal image of a pseudogestational sac, which represents a collection of fluid within the decidualized endometrial cavity

some ectopic pregnancies. The pseudogestational sac represents an accumulation of fluid or blood within the decidualized endometrium (Figure 14.9). In patients with minimal peritoneal findings, serial quantitative β-hCG titers and repeat transvaginal scans at 48–72-h intervals are required to make the diagnosis.

The diagnosis of complete abortion can be made by ultrasound when the uterine cavity is empty and one of the following criteria is fulfilled:

(1) The uterine cavity appears empty and serial β-hCG quantitative titers are rapidly falling towards negative. Initially, the titers should be taken at 48-h intervals;

(2) An intrauterine pregnancy had been demonstrated on an earlier ultrasound, but the uterine cavity is now empty;

(3) Pathology reveals the presence of products of conception.

Failure to meet any of these criteria can lead to the diagnosis of ectopic pregnancy being missed. The rare phenomenon of heterotopic pregnancy, which is becoming more common with assisted reproduction, should not be forgotten.

Functional and hemorrhagic ovarian cysts

Functional cysts are extremely common in menstrual-age women. Approximately 15% of asymptomatic menstrual-age women will have a cyst > 2.5 cm. when screened[6,7]. Most functional cysts appear to be predominantly cystic and are usually < 6 cm in diameter. The cysts usually disappear spontaneously after 1–2 menstrual cycles with or without the use of contraception pills[8].

Hemorrhagic cysts vary widely in echo patterns. They may be filled with uniform low-level internal echoes, thereby mimicking the pattern typically associated with endometriomas (Figures 14.10–14.13)[9]. They may contain areas of resorbing or retracting clot and mimic the appearance of both benign or malignant neoplasms[10]. Fortunately, most hemorrhagic cysts disappear spontaneously within 1–2 menstrual cycles. Color Doppler is also a powerful tool

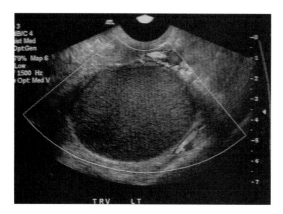

Figure 14.10 Transvaginal image of an endometrioma. Approximately 60–70% of endometriotic cysts are filled with low-level echoes, a pattern which is also seen in hemorrhagic cysts and abscesses

Figure 14.11 Transvaginal image of a resolving hemorrhagic corpus luteum shows a cribriform pattern of low-level echoes within the cyst. These masses usually spontaneously resolve within 4–8 weeks

Figure 14.12 Transvaginal image of a resolving hemorrhagic corpus luteum showing low-level internal echoes within the cyst

Figure 14.13 Transvaginal image of a complex mass with a papillary-like internal projection. Pathology revealed a corpus luteum; the echogenic material (arrow) was clotted blood. A cystic teratoma or papillary adenocarcinoma may present an identical image

because almost all malignant tumors will display solid regions or excrescences with central pulsatile vascular flow[11,12]. Clots do not display pulsatile flow, and corporea lutea can usually be identified by peripheral vasculature flow. Since functionals cysts, hemorrhagic cysts and endometriomas make up 75–80% of ovarian masses seen in the premenopause, it is critical that the gynecologist be familiar with the character-istic ultrasound appearance of these cysts and their management.

Ovarian neoplasms

Ultrasound attributes associated with a high probability of benign disease include a mass

Figure 14.14 Transabdominal image showing a densely echogenic cystic teratoma

Figure 14.15 Transvaginal image of a cystic teratoma with a large cystic component and a papillary-like projection with posterior shadowing. The echo pattern of cystic teratomas is frequently complex and can make differentiation from malignant tumors difficult

that is < 8 cm or cystic, minimally septated or with no solid areas[13]. However, in premenopausal women, dermoid cysts are the exception to these characteristics. Some workers believe that these masses can be preoperatively identified by their characteristic dense echogenicity and posterior shadowing (Figures 14.14 and 14.15)[14,15]. A higher index for suspected ovarian malignancy should be considered if a neoplasm is found in a postmenopausal woman; a mass > 8 cm, multiseptations and solid areas within a neoplasm are all associated with a higher risk of malignancy (Figures 14.16 and 14.17). Review of multiple different logistic regression series has shown there are two most important characteristics for differentiating malignant from benign disease. The first is the presence or absence of solid elements. The second is the presence or absence of central pulsatile flow within these solid elements[11,12]. The role of arbitrary velocimetry cut-off values remains hotly debated.

The inexperienced sonologist is advised to seek second opinions when an adnexal mass is found during an ultrasound examination although, even with years of ultrasound experience, it is an imperfect art.

Figure 14.16 A poorly differentiated stage III adenocarcinoma in a menopausal women. The tumor contains multilocular areas as well as solid elements with central vascular flow on Doppler

In postmenopausal women, the presence of a cystic mass < 6 cm does not necessarily indicate that the patient requires surgery (Figure 14.18). Such a finding is seen in 2–3% of postmenopausal women[16] and, in many centers, these women have been followed by repeat examination and measurement of CA-125 tumor marker levels at

Figure 14.17 A stage III poorly differentiated adenocarcinoma of the ovary. The neoplasm is solid with abnormal central flow

Figure 14.18 Transvaginal image of a thin-walled 4.5-cm cyst in a postmenopausal woman shows no septations, solid areas or neovascularization

6-month intervals; surgery is performed only if clinically indicated.

Dysfunctional bleeding

Transvaginal ultrasonography allows rapid evaluation of uterine size, contour and cavity. The presence of myomas is generally easily established as the echo density and capsules of these tumors usually differ markedly from those of normal uterine tissue[17]. Particular attention should be paid to centrally located leiomyomas which may be submucous or to leiomyomas that appear to impinge on the cavity of the uterus, as these tumors are a major cause of abnormal uterine bleeding. A secretory endometrium can aid in the demarcation of submucous leiomyomas. Color and power Doppler can also be used to identify 'feeder vessels' entering space-occupying lesions of the cavity[18] (Figures 14.19–14.21).

Adenomyosis

The clinician should also remember that adenomyosis can cause heavy irregular periods,

Figure 14.19 A 2.5 cm submucous leiomyoma outlined by a secretory endometrium. Infusion was deferred since minimal myometrial penetration was clearly documented

but is frequently not obvious on transvaginal scanning. The best clues are diffuse uterine enlargement, absence of myoma-like echoes and, occasionally, visualization of glandular spaces in the uterine wall. Magnetic resonance imaging (MRI) appears to be more accurate than transvaginal ultrasound in identifying adenomyosis. In many cases it may be necessary to perform a sonohysterogram to define better intracavitary lesions[19].

Figure 14.20 A single feeder vessel is noted within an echogenic endometrium using Doppler. Pathology revealed an endometrial polyp

Figure 14.21 Another enometrial polyp with a feeder vessel.

Figure 14.22 A 2-D sonohysterogram identifies a 5 × 3 mm. Endometrial polyp

Figure 14.23 A 2-D sonohysterogram clearly demarcates a posterior lower uterine segment leiomyoma. Power Doppler reveals deep myometrial penetration

Sonohysterography

Sonohysterography in the office frequently may provide improved visualization of the uterine cavity. Sonohysterography is particularly useful in identifying small polyps and in assessing the size and degree of myometrial penetration of submucous leiomyomas[20,21] (Figures 14.22 and 14.23). The technique is easily learned and simply involves instillation of sterile saline while scanning. Many differ-

ent catheters have been used. It is our preference to use catheters with a small balloon to prevent leakage of fluid during the study. The elliptosphere catheter (Ackrad Laboratories) can be placed in the cervix or serially deflated to visualize better the lower aspect of the cavity. Care should be taken not to perform sonohysterograms in women who are potentially pregnant. Premedication with non-steroidal anti-inflammatory agents is strongly recommended. Sceening for and

Figure 14.24 A 3-D coronal image using sonohysterography clearly demonstates two endometrial polyps

Figure 14.25 A 3-D coronal image using sonohysterography with a labelled endometrial polyp and and a intramural leiomyoma

history of pelvic inflammatory disease should be obtained to avoid the risk of pelvic peritonitis. 3-D imaging and Doppler mapping are very useful adjuncts to sonohysterography.[22,23] (Figures 14.24–14.26)

Failure to map properly submucous leiomyomas can result in poor case selection and outcome. For the hysteroscopic surgeon to be successful, the depth of penetration of the submucous leiomyoma in the uterine walls must be appreciated. Serious consideration should be given to MRI with contrast when ultrasound is not satisfactory.

Figure 14.26 A 3-D coronal image from a sonohysterogram demonstates two minimally penetrating submucous leiomyomas

Postmenopausal bleeding

Although endometrial biopsy remains the gold standard for evaluation of postmenopausal bleeding, TVS can be used to assess the risk for endometrial malignancy in these patients. Karlsson and colleagues[24] studied a large series of 1168 women with postmenopausal bleeding, 114 of whom had endometrial cancer, and demonstrated that the endometrial stripe should be " 4 mm in postmenopausal women not receiving hormone replacement therapy (HRT). A recent

consensus report has suggested that either endometrial biopsy or measurement of endometrial thickness is satisfactory for the evaluation of menopausal bleeding[25]. In a study by Zalud and co-workers[26] in postmenopausal women taking continuous HRT (conjugated estrogens (Premarin® 0.625 mg) and medroxyprogesterone acetate (Provera® 2.5 mg daily), the investigators found that the average ± 1 standard deviation endometrial thickness was 7.6 ± 2.6 mm. Bonilla-Musoles and colleagues, using a different

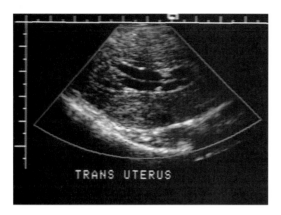

Figure 14.27 A tamoxifen-stimulated endometrial polyp

Figure 14.28 A tamoxifen-stimulated hemorrhagic cyst

form of continuous HRT regimen (Estraderm TTS® (patch) and Provera 2.5 mg) found an average endometrial thickness of 4.2 mm (range 0–14 mm). These investigators also reported an average endometrial thickness of 6.6 mm (range 2–15 mm) with sequential therapy (Estraderm TTS and Provera 10 mg on days 17–28 of the cycle)[27]. Lin and co-workers demonstrated an average endometrial stripe of 6 ± 3.9 mm (range 0.1–17 mm) in women taking cyclical therapy (Premarin 0.625–1.25 mg on cycle days 1–25 and Provera 5 or 10 mg on the last 10–13 days of estrogen therapy)[28]. It has not been established in the literature whether it is safe to use a > 5 mm endometrial thickness cut-off point in women with irregular post-menopausal bleeding receiving HRT.

Tamoxifen effects

Tamoxifen can lead to thickening of the endometrium in both pre- and post-menopausal women. Large endometrial polyps may be seen with use of this medication (Figure 14.27). The endometrial stripe

may be difficult to measure in post-menopausal women owing to the appearance of subepithelial lucencies. In the presence of irregular bleeding, a sonohysterogram or hysteroscopy in addition to biopsy may be required to evaluate these patients. Tamoxifen can also lead to hyperstimulation of the ovary, particularly in premenopausal patients (Figure 14.28).

Uterine anomalies

3-D office ultrasound without infusion now provides an excellent low-cost alternative to the use of endoscopy, MRI and hysterography in the evaluation of uterine anomalies. The technique is particularly powerful in differentiating an arcuate from a septate uterus. The uterine fundus can be easily evaluated and thick septa differentiated from bicornuate uteri[29,30] (Figures 14.29 and 14.30).

SUMMARY

Transvaginal ultrasound (TVS) is a powerful tool that all gynecologists should be

Figure 14.29 A 3-D study with coronal reconstruction without infusion of a bicornuate uterus

Figure 14.30 A 3-D study without infusion using coronal reconstuction of a complete uterine septum

comfortable using. Clearly, for the evaluation of abnormalities of early pregnancy, TVS is indispensable. TVS is also an important initial triage step in the evaluation of both pre- and postmenopausal bleeding, since it allows for the identification of thickened endometrium and space-occupying lesions. The addition of sonohysterography, Doppler mapping and 3-D imaging can help in proper case selection for hysteroscopic surgery. TVS also allows for immediate evaluation of suspect adnexal masses in the office setting. For those not performing their own TVS procedures, hopefully this chapter will serve as encouragement to learn and master this powerful diagnostic tool.

REFERENCES

1. Timor-Tritsch IE, Yeh MN, Peisner DB, *et al.* The use of transvaginal sonography in the diagnosis of ectopic pregnancy. *Am J Obstet Gynecol* 1989;161:157–61

2. Warren WB, Timor-Tritsch IE, Peisner DB, *et al.* Dating the early pregnancy by sequential appearance of embryonic structures. *Am J Obstet Gynecol* 1989;161:747–53

3. American College of Obstetrics and Gynecology. Ectopic pregnancy. *ACOG Tech Bull* 1990;December (150)

4. Rempen A. Diagnosis of viability in early pregnancy with vaginal sonography. *J Ultrasound Med* 1990;9:711–16

5. Pennell RG, Needleman L, Pajak T, *et al.* Prospective comparison of vaginal and abdominal sonography in normal early pregnancy. *J Ultrasound Med* 1991;10:63–7

6. Borgfeldt C, Andolf E. Transvaginal sonographic findings in a random sample of women 25–40 years old. *Ultrasound Obstet Gynecol* 1999;13:345–9

7. Shulman H, Conway C, Zalud I, *et al.* Prevalence in a volunteer population of pelvic cancer detected with transvaginal ultrasound and color Doppler. *Ultrasound Obstet Gynecol* 1994;4:414–20

8. Steinkampf MP, Hammond KR, Blackwell RE. Hormonal treatment of functional ovarian cysts: a randomized prospective study. *Fertil Steril* 1990;54:775

9. Cohen L, Valle RF, Sabbagha RE. A comparison of the preoperative ultrasound images of surgically proven endometriomas scanned by both transabdominal and transvaginal techniques. *J Gynecol Surg* 1995;11:27–32

10. Jain KA. Sonographic spectrum of hemorrhagic ovarian cysts. *J Ultrasound Med* 2002;21:879–86

11. Timmerman D, Bourne TH, Tailor A, *et al.* A comparison of methods for preoperative discrimination between malignant and benign masses. The development of a new logistic regression model. *Am J Obstet Gynecol* 1999;181:57–65

12. Schelling M, Braun M, Kuhn W, *et al.* Combined transvaginal B-mode and color Doppler sonography for differential diagnosis of ovarian tumors: results of a multivariate logistic regression analysis. *Gynecol Oncol* 2000;77:78–86

13. Maiman M, Seltzer V, Boyce J. Laparoscopic excision of ovarian masses subsequently found to be malignant. *Obstet Gynecol* 1991;77:563–6

14. Mais V, Guerriero S, Ajossa S, *et al.* Trans-vaginal ultrasonography in the diagnosis of cystic teratoma. *Obstet Gynecol* 1995;85:48–52

15. Cohen L, Sabbagha R. Echo patterns of benign cystic teratomas by transvaginal ultrasound. *Ultrasound Obstet Gynecol* 1993;3:120–3

16. Bailley C, Ueland F, Land G, *et al.* The malignant potential of small cystic ovarian tumors in women over 50 years of age. *Gynecol Oncol* 1998;69:3–7

17. Fedele L, Bianchi S, Dorta M, *et al.* Transvaginal sonography versus hysteros-copy in the diagnosis of uterine submucous myomas. *Obstet Gynecol* 1991;77:745

18. Fleischer AC, Shappell HW. *Color Doppler sono-hysterography of endometrial polyps and submucous fibroids. J Ultrasound Med* 2003;22:601–4

19. Deuholm M, Lundorf E, Hansen ES, *et al.* Magnetic resonance imaging and transvaginal ultrasonography for diagnosis of adenomyosis. *Fertil Steril* 2001:76:588–94

20. Cohen LS, Valle RF. Role of vaginal sonography and hysterosonography in the endoscopic treatment of uterine myomas. *Fertil Steril* 2000;73:197–204

21. Deuholm M, Forman A, Jensen ML, *et al.* Transvaginal sonography combined with saline contrast sonohysterography in evaluating the uterine cavity. *Ultrasound Obstet Gynecol* 2001;18:54–61

22. Cohen LS, Buckley A, Valle RF. The role of three-dimensional transvaginal ultrasound in the evaluation of premenopausal abnormal uterine bleeding. *J Gynecol Surg* 2000; 16:69–77

23. Lev-Toaff AS, Pinheiro LW, Bega G *et al.* Three-dimensional multiplanar sonohysterography. *J Ultrasound Med* 2001;20:295–306

24. Karlsson B, Granberg S, Wikland M, *et al.* Transvaginal ultrasonography of the endometrium in women with postmenopausal bleeding. A Nordic multicenter study. *Am J Obstet Gynecol* 1995;172:1488–94

25. Goldstein RB, Bree RL, Benacerraf BB, *et al.* Evaluation of women with postmenopausal bleeding. Society of Radiologists in Ultrasound-Sponsored Consensus Conference. *J Ultasound Med* 2001;20: 1025–36

26. Zalud I, Conway C, Schulmann H, Trinca D. Endometrial and myometrial thickness and uterine blood flow in postmenopausal women: the influence of hormone replacement and age. *J Ultrasound Med* 1993;12:737–41

27. Bonilla-Musoles F, Ballester MJ, Marti M, *et al.* Transvaginal colour Doppler assessment of endometrial status in normal postmenopausal women: the effect of hormone replacement therapy. *J Ultrasound Med* 1995;14:503–7

28. Lin M, Gosink B, Wolf S, *et al.* Endometrial thickness after menopause: effect of hormone replacement. *Radiology* 1991;180:427–32

29. Jurkovic D, Geipel A, Gruboeck K, *et al.* Three-dimensional ultrasound for the assessment of uterine anatomy and detection of congenital anomalies: a comparison with hysterosalpingography and two-dimensional sonography. *Ultrasound Obstet Gynecol* 1995;5:233–7

30. Woelfer B, Salim R, Banerjee S, *et al.* Reproductive outcomes in women with congenital uterine anomalies detected by three-dimensional ultrasound screening. *Obstet Gynecol* 2001;98:1099–103

15

Computed tomography and magnetic resonance imaging in gynecology

Paul Nikolaidis and Frederick L. Hoff

Imaging of the female pelvis is dominated by ultrasonography. Ultrasound has three principal advantages over other modalities: real-time capability, lack of ionizing radiation and relative low cost. Ultrasound is the only imaging modality required in many clinical situations. However, it is incumbent upon the gynecologist to be comfortable reviewing and be cognizant of the advantages and disadvantages of computed tomography (CT) and magnetic resonance imaging (MRI). There are settings in which CT or MRI can provide additional or unique information that is helpful to the gynecologist. In addition, CTs and MRIs ordered in the evaluation of vague or confusing symptoms may indicate an unsuspected gynecological origin of the symptoms. For these reasons, the gynecologist should not only know when these modalities may be helpful, but should also have a working knowledge of the basics of the procedures and the significance of the findings. This chapter covers the more frequently encountered abnormalities as well as those situations in which CT and MRI can provide valuable information to the clinician.

COMPUTED TOMOGRAPHY

Technique

Conventional CT scanners have an X-ray tube and a bank of detectors mounted on a rotating gantry. The gantry rotates once around the stationary patient to create a digitized cross-sectional axial image. Beginning in the early 1990s, helical and then multidetector helical CT revolutionized the modality, creating many new applications and improving upon older ones. In helical CT, the X-ray tube and detectors are mounted on a slip ring that can rotate continuously as the patient moves through the machine, allowing rapid acquisition of data. Multidetector helical CT units still use one X-ray tube but have multiple rows of detector elements, obtaining from two to 64 sets of data with each rotation. This has allowed a progressive decrease in slice thickness and scans that can be completed well within a single breath-hold. The acquisition of multiple thin, overlapped images during a single breath-hold has allowed the routine use of sagittal and coronal image reconstructions.

Contrast agents are used in CT to alter the density of adjacent structures. Oral contrast (usually a solution of dilute barium) is nearly always indicated, primarily to prevent a bowel loop from mimicking a cystic adnexal abnormality or adenopathy. Similarly, rectal contrast can distend the rectum and colon to differentiate better pelvic involvement of a tumor or infection. Intravenous iodine-based contrast is also helpful in identifying vascular structures and distinguishing solid masses from fluid.

Figure 15.1 Normal computed tomography (CT) of the pelvis. (a) Axial CT through the pelvis after administration of intravenous contrast. The uterus (curved arrow) is located in the mid-pelvis; the central area of low density represents the endometrium (e). The ovaries are seen laterally (arrowheads). The left ureter is well visualized, being filled with dense contrast (open arrow). (b) An image taken more caudally (same patient as in (a) demonstrates the cervix (curved arrow) and endocervical canal (arrow). The round ligaments (arrowheads) are noted anteriorly. (c) The uterus (U) and broad ligaments (long arrows) are well outlined by the adjacent ascites that fills the pelvis. The external (open arrows) and internal (arrowheads) iliac vessels are also seen

Normal pelvic CT anatomy

The uterus is routinely visualized as a well-defined muscle-density structure (Figure 15.1a); however, the amount of useful information is dependent on the uterine position. The endometrium is slightly lower in density than the adjacent myometrium. The cervix is similar in density to the uterus (Figure 15.1b) and is difficult to differentiate from the vaginal fornices surrounding it. Distally, the vagina is seen as a collapsed H-shaped structure. The ovaries appear as heterogeneous structures of soft tissue and fluid density lying lateral to the uterus (Figure 15.1a). The normal Fallopian tubes

and broad ligaments are not well visualized unless surrounded by ascites (Figure 15.1c). The round ligaments may occasionally be identified (Figure 15.1b).

The surrounding structures of the pelvis are well demonstrated by CT. The common, external and internal iliac arteries and veins are seen in nearly all patients (Figure 15.1c). They are easily located knowing their characteristic locations adjacent to the psoas, iliopsoas and obturator internus muscles. The ureter crosses anterior to the iliac artery bifurcation and then courses medially at the level of the sciatic foramen; it can be best demonstrated if filled with contrast material (Figure 15.1a). Normal lymph nodes appear as soft-tissue-density structures adjacent to the pelvic vessels less than 1 cm in short-axis dimension.

INDICATIONS FOR PELVIC CT

There are relatively few specific indications for CT of the female genital tract. Many clinical situations are better evaluated by other means, such as ultrasound and laparoscopy. However, CT can be used to evaluate inflammatory diseases, identify pelvic masses and stage malignancies. Patients who present with acute pain and fever may have inflammatory conditions such as appendicitis, diverticulitis, inflammatory bowel disease or pelvic inflammatory disease. Because clinically these conditions may overlap, CT can be useful in their evaluation, particularly when results of ultrasound are normal or equivocal. Postoperative patients with possible abscesses are also good candidates for CT; in such patients, ultrasound may often be limited by pain and associated ileus.

FINDINGS ON PELVIC CT

Uterine leiomyoma

Uterine leiomyomas are typically hypodense or isodense with the surrounding myometrium (Figure 15.2). Although they are occasionally seen as well-defined masses, the most common finding is uterine enlargement and a deformed contour. On occasion, it may be difficult to differentiate between a centrally located leiomyoma and endometrial abnormality. The presence of calcification can make identification easier, although only a minority contain calcium.

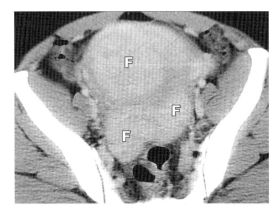

Figure 15.2 Uterine leiomyoma. Helical CT through the pelvis obtained during bolus administration of intravenous contrast shows three discrete enhancing uterine fibroids (F)

Adnexal findings

Mature teratoma (dermoid cyst)

Most mature teratomas are well-defined masses (Figure 15.3) that often contain multiple elements, including lipid and calcification. A specific diagnosis can be made in up to 98% of cases[1].

Ovarian tumor

Ovarian epithelial tumors generally have both low-density fluid and high-density soft-tissue components (Figure 15.4). These findings in an adnexal mass on CT are non-specific; malignant masses are not reliably differentiated from benign masses, although the presence of wall thickening, thickened septations, papillary projections and solid components all suggest malignancy. More important is the capability preoperatively to identify invasion (Figure 15.5), hydronephrosis, ascites, peritoneal implants and pleural effusions. CT has a reported staging accuracy of 70–90% and may be helpful in presurgical planning[2].

147

Figure 15.3 Ovarian dermoid. CT reveals a small left adnexal mass (arrowheads) containing areas of low-density fat and high-density calcium (arrow). This is essentially diagnostic of a dermoid. The uterus (U) and right ovary (R) are normal

Figure 15.4 Ovarian serous cystadenoma. CT reveals a lobulated mass (arrows) centrally in the pelvis. The mass is predominantly fluid in density but contains multiple thick and thin septa (arrowheads). Although non-specific, the presence of thickened septations raises the possibility of malignancy. This proved to be a serous cystadenoma on resection

Tubo-ovarian abscess

Abscesses on CT are identified as low-density fluid collections that often have an enhanced, thick wall (Figure 15.6). Associated findings of pelvic inflammatory disease include an increased density in the adjacent fat ('fat stranding') and obscuration of the normal fascial planes, as well as thickening of the uterosacral ligaments, Fallopian tubes or adjacent structures. Although non-specific, these findings are highly suggestive in the appropriate clinical setting. CT is particularly useful for atypical cases or when ultrasound is equivocal[3].

Hydro/hemato/pyosalpinx

Hydrosalpinx should be suspected whenever a tubular mass is seen in the adnexa on CT (Figure 15.7). As the dilated Fallopian tube is usually serpiginous, on any single image the abnormality may appear to represent a cyst or multiple cysts; by viewing multiple adjacent images or coronal reformatted images one can determine whether these join to form a tubular structure. In general, it is difficult to differentiate hydro-, pyo- and hematosalpinx on the basis of CT findings alone. Clinical history and the presence of adjacent abnormalities may help to differentiate these entities.

Miscellaneous findings

Appendicitis

Helical CT is an excellent test in the diagnosis of appendicitis. The use of preoperative CT in suspected cases of appendicitis is nearly routine in many centers and has been credited with decreasing negative laparotomy rates, perforation rates, severity of pathological findings and hospital stays[4]. The appendix is identified as a blind-ending tubular structure arising from the cecum, and is abnormal if there is wall thickening, enlargement (greater than

Figure 15.5 Ovarian mucinous cystadenocarcinoma. CT showing a large pelvic mass with predominately solid (arrow) components and only a few cystic (curved arrow) areas. The mass has invaded the sigmoid colon (short arrow). The large solid component indicates this is probably a malignant mass; its invasive nature confirms it

Figure 15.6 Tubo-ovarian abscess. CT reveals a left adnexal thick-walled fluid collection (arrow); the patient had clinical symptoms of pelvic inflammatory disease not responding to antibiotics. This proved to be a tubo-ovarian abscess. Also labeled are the bladder (curved arrow) and uterus (U), which is displaced to the left by the abscess

Figure 15.7 Hematosalpinx. (a) Post-contrast CT image shows a fluid-density tubular structure (arrowheads) in the left adnexa. (b) A second image obtained 2 cm caudal to (a), also shows the tubular structure as well as two uterine cornua (labeled R and L). The left horn (L) is distended by low-density material. This was confirmed at surgery to be a hematosalpinx and hematometra secondary to a unicornuate uterus with a non-communicating left remnant

6 mm diameter) or increased density in the periappendiceal fat (Figure 15.8). CT has been reported to have an accuracy of nearly 98% with a 99% negative predictive value in one large 5-year retrospective review[5].

Postoperative studies

The appearance of a postoperative abscess is similar to that of a tubo-ovarian abscess, although the location is more variable. CT has advantages over ultrasound particularly in identifying intraloop abscesses and when

Figure 15.8 Appendicitis. CT showing an enlarged appendix (arrow) with a thickened, abnormally enhancing wall; inflammatory changes can be seen in the adjacent fat. These findings are diagnostic of acute appendicitis

Figure 15.9 Postoperative fistula. A CT in a patient status post-hysterectomy with a suspected urinary fistula to the vagina. A tampon was placed in the vagina and narrow slices were obtained after administration of intravenous contrast. A thin fistula between the left ureter and vagina can be seen; the tampon is high in density due to the enhanced urine it has absorbed

ultrasound is hindered by patient pain and bowel gas associated with postoperative ileus. Fistulas (Figure 15.9) and other abnormalities may also be demonstrated.

Adenopathy

Lymph nodes are identified as well-defined soft-tissue-density structures adjacent to the pelvic vasculature. The obturator nodes are particularly important because they are a common site of first spread of many pelvic tumors. Involvement by tumor can be predicted on the basis of size: a short-axis diameter > 15 mm is considered to be abnormal, whereas those that are 11–14 mm are considered indeterminate[6].

MAGNETIC RESONANCE IMAGING

Technique

Although a lengthy explanation of the physics of MRI is beyond the scope of this chapter, a brief explanation will allow the gynecologist to understand the terminology used to describe the findings with these studies. MRI uses a static magnetic field to align protons within the body. A short burst of electromagnetic radiation in the radiowave frequency range is then applied to disturb the aligned protons from the baseline state. As the protons within the patient relax back to baseline, they in turn emit electromagnetic radiation; antennae within the MRI unit detect these radiowaves coming from the patient. This released energy forms the basis of the image and the amount of signal detected is displayed on a gray scale. Differences in the amount of signal emanating from tissues are due to three factors: T1 relaxation time, T2 relaxation time and the density of free protons. These factors are intrinsic to a tissue and are constant. Variations in the way a particular sequence excites the tissue will change the relative effect that each of these three factors has on the final image.

Accordingly, sequences that accentuate the effects of the T1 relaxation time are referred to as 'T1-weighted sequences', and those that accentuate the T2 relaxation time are called 'T2-weighted sequences'. In evaluating the uterus, T2-weighted images are the most helpful. In general, however, the signal intensity of a structure as determined on several different sequences is needed to characterize the structure fully.

Gadolinium is attached to a complex molecule (for safety purposes) and used as an intravenous contrast agent similar to the iodinated contrast agents used in CT. Regions enhanced with gadolinium are high in signal (bright) on appropriate sequences. In general, gadolinium agents are considerably safer than iodinated agents and are associated with a much lower incidence of allergic reactions and renal complications. There are a number of relative and absolute contraindications to the use of MRI, but these are beyond the scope of this chapter. Most centers screen each patient for such contraindications both at the time of making an appointment and immediately before the study is carried out.

NORMAL PELVIC ANATOMY ON MRI

The uterus is well demonstrated on MRI (Figure 15.10). As with ultrasonography, the appearance of the uterus varies through the menstrual cycle. Three zones or layers are identified: the myometrium, the junctional zone and the endometrium. The zonal anatomy is best identified on T2-weighted images. The signal intensity of the myometrium changes according to the phase of the menstrual cycle, increasing during the secretory phase due to increased fluid content. The middle layer, or junctional zone, has low signal intensity and represents the longitudinally oriented smooth muscle of the basal layer of the myometrium[7]. Its appearance is of a thin low-signal-intensity line between the high-signal endometrium and intermediate-signal myometrium, averaging 5 mm in thickness. This layer does not change during the menstrual cycle, but may become attenuated in the menopause. The endometrium is high in signal on T2-weighted images and becomes progressively thicker through the menstrual cycle. The endometrium is measured on sagittal T2-weighted images through the middle portion of the uterus, including both layers. In premenopausal women, it ranges in thickness from 3 to 10 mm, whereas in postmenopausal women who are not taking exogenous hormones, it should be no thicker than 4 mm[8].

The cervix is predominantly low in signal intensity on T2-weighted images due to its dense fibrous stroma. Centrally located is a thin high-signal-intensity stripe representing the endocervix with glandular fluid and mucus. The vagina is best visualized on axial T2-weighted images. A H-shaped high-signal-intensity line represents the collapsed mucosa and any fluid or secretions within the vagina. This is surrounded by the intermediate- to low-signal-intensity muscular wall and the high-signal-intensity perivaginal venous plexus. The urethra can be identified as a round structure lying immediately anterior to the vagina and also surrounded by the venous plexus. The normal ovaries are reliably identified on MRI. They are usually most easily found on T2-weighted sequences as oval-shaped structures with multiple, small, high-signal-intensity follicles.

Figure 15.10 Normal magnetic resonance imagine (MRI) of the pelvis. (a) Short-axis T2-weighted MRI of the anteverted uterus (coronal to the patient) shows that the myometrium has intermediate signal intensity (short arrow) and the endometrium (long arrow) has high signal intensity; the low-signal junctional zone is visualized between the two. The bladder is noted caudal to the uterus (curved arrow); fluid (urine) is bright on T2-weighted images. (b) Sagittal midline MRI reveals an anteflexed uterus (arrow) with normal zonal anatomy. The bladder (B) is anterior and air is seen in the sigmoid colon (*). (c) Sagittal MRI obtained laterally shows a normal ovary (arrowheads) with multiple high-signal follicles

INDICATIONS FOR PELVIC MRI

The routine use of MRI to evaluate disease of the female pelvis has been limited, despite the fact that there are several conditions that are better demonstrated by MRI than by any other imaging modality. These conditions include congenital uterine anomalies, leiomyomas and adenomyosis. Limited access, perceived cost differentials and lack of physician awareness may account for some of the underuse of MRI[9]. Indeed, there is some evidence that the use of MRI may decrease medical costs. Schwartz and colleagues have examined the impact of MRI studies of the female pelvis on treatment decisions and net cost of treatment[10]. Their results demonstrated that treatment plans after the use of MRI included fewer operations and an increased use of less invasive surgery, representing overall savings in the treatment of the 69 women in their sample. Similarly, the use of MRI in the staging and monitoring of cervical and endometrial carcinoma is sporadic, despite evidence that preoperative staging of clinical stage Ib cervical carcinoma is helpful and cost-effective[11].

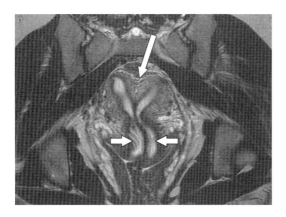

Figure 15.11 Congenital anomaly, uterus didelphys. A long-axis T2-weighted MR image of the uterus demonstrates two separate uterine horns with no intervening myometrium (long arrow). Two separate cervices are also present (arrows)

Figure 15.12 Congenital anomaly, septate uterus. A long-axis T2-weighted MR image of the uterus demonstrates a distinct septum extending to the lower uterine segment (arrow). There is a convex fundal contour (arrowheads), with no fundal indentation, as would be seen in a bicornuate uterus

FINDINGS ON PELVIC MRI

Uterus

Congenital anomalies

MRI is an excellent modality for demonstrating the full spectrum of congenital uterine anomalies. The multiplanar ability of MRI allows the routine display of coronal long-axis images of the uterus. MRI provides excellent visualization of both the endometrium and myometrium, combining, in one study, the advantages of both hysterosalpingography and ultrasonography. In a study of 26 patients with Müllerian duct anomalies, MRI was 100% accurate in the diagnoses, whereas ultrasound was 92% accurate and hystero-salpingog-raphy only 16% accurate[12]. Of particular value is the accuracy of MRI in differentiating a septate uterus that can be treated through the hysteroscope from the bicornuate uterus that cannot (Figures 15.11 and 15.12). MRI alone may be able to provide an accurate and adequate preoperative assessment in patients with uterine and vaginal septa. MRI may also reliably diagnose other Müllerian duct anomalies, such as a unicornuate uterus (Figure 15.13); the presence of a clinically suspected rudimentary horn may also be confirmed[13]. Finally, the presence of other associated genitourinary tract anomalies such as unilateral renal agenesis may be assessed by utilizing a large field-of-view coronal or sagittal sequence.

Leiomyoma

Transvaginal ultrasound has been reported to be as effective as MRI for detection of uterine leiomyomas, but MRI outperforms transvaginal ultrasound in preoperative evaluation of location, number and size of leiomyomas[14]. On MRI, leiomyomas usually appear as sharply marginated masses that typically have lower signal intensity than the myometrium on T2-weighted images[15]. Use of imaging planes in both the short and

Figure 15.13 Congenital anomaly, unicornuate uterus. A long-axis T2-weighted MR image of the uterus demonstrates a single uterine horn extending to the left of midline (arrow). There is a non-communicating rudimentary horn (H)

Figure 15.14 Submucosal leiomyoma. Axial (a) and sagittal (b) T2-weighted MR images of the uterus in the same patient show a rounded hypointense submucosal leiomyoma (L) projecting into the hyperintense endometrial cavity. Note the normal-appearing ovaries (arrows) and bladder (B)

the long axis of the uterus provides sufficient information to assign specific locations as well as to differentiate submucosal, intramural and subserosal tumors (Figures 15.14 and 15.15). Also, MRI readily differentiates pedunculated submucosal leiomyomas from other solid pelvic masses when ultrasound is indeterminate.

MRI can also identify complications within leiomyomas. Some leiomyomas have areas of high signal intensity on T2-weighted images that may represent either degeneration or cellularity[16]. Red degeneration of a leiomyoma may have the specific appearance of a hyperintense rim on T1-weighted images that is hypointense on T2-weighted images; this may be useful in the evaluation of symptomatic patients. As with ultrasound and CT, MRI cannot identify sarcomatous degeneration within a leiomyoma.

With the recent advent of uterine artery embolization as an alternative to hysterectomy in women with symptomatic leiomyomas, MRI has been proved highly useful in pre- and post-embolization evaluation (Figure 15.16)[17].

Adenomyosis

Adenomyosis is a process in which endometrial glands and stroma are present deep within the myometrium. Adenomyosis can be difficult to diagnose clinically, ultrasonographically or invasively. MRI is very sensitive in the detection of this condition, superior to endovaginal ultrasound (Figure 15.17). Findings on MRI include focal or diffuse junctional zone thickness over 10 mm, or a low-signal-intensity myometrial mass with indistinct margins on T2-weighted images[18,19]. Furthermore, high-signal foci

Figure 15.15 Multiple uterine leiomyomas. Coronal (a) and sagittal (b) T2-weighted MR images of the uterus in the same patient demonstrate several rounded hypointense intramural leiomyomas (L) as well as an anterior subserosal leiomyoma (SL). Note the thin hyperintense endometrium (arrow)

Figure 15.16 Uterine artery embolization. Sagittal T1-weighted fat-saturated post-gadolinium MR images demonstrating a uterine leiomyoma pre- and post-uterine artery embolization. (a) Pre-embolization scan: the leiomyoma (arrow) demonstrates intense enhancement. (b) Post-embolization scan: 5 weeks after embolization there is almost no contrast enhancement of this leiomyoma (arrow), indicating a successful uterine artery embolization procedure. The leiomyoma is expected to decrease further in size over the next few months

within the low-intensity myometrium are often seen on T2-weighted sequences. These T2-bright foci are thought to represent endometrial tissue, endometrial cysts or hemorrhagic foci[20]. Particularly helpful is the differentiation between adenomyosis and leiomyomas in patients presenting with an enlarged uterus; this is easily accomplished by MRI[18]. Togashi and colleagues examined 93 women with uterine enlargement prospectively; of the 71 who had leiomyomas and the 16 with adenomyosis, all but one were correctly diagnosed by MRI[21].

Cervix

Cervical tumors

The potential role of MRI is not in the diagnosis of cervical carcinoma, but rather in

Figure 15.17 Adenomyosis. Sagittal T2-weighted MRI demonstrates a diffusely widened junctional zone containing multiple punctate high-intensity foci (arrows). Both findings are diagnostic of adenomyosis. This is in contrast to the normal junctional zone depicted in Figure 15.10. Also note the bright endometrium (e), collapsed bladder (curved arrow) and small amount of free fluid (f), which is probably physiological

Figure 15.18 Cervical tumor. Sagittal T1-weighted fat-saturated post-gadolinium MRI showing a large high-signal-intensity mass (arrowheads) arising from the cervix, enlarging the vagina as well as extending into the endometrial cavity (arrow). This proved to be a malignant mixed Müllerian tumor with predominant sarcomatous elements. The bladder (B) is seen anteriorly

the improvement of its staging. Although there is at present no general acceptance of a role for MRI in this process, MRI has been demonstrated to be both useful and cost-effective in the preoperative evaluation of stage Ib disease, if the tumor is greater than 2 cm in size or endocervical in location[11,22]. MRI has also been demonstrated to be superior for monitoring treatment response and for evaluating recurrent disease[23]. Cervical carcinoma is most commonly seen as a well-defined soft-tissue-enhancing mass on MRI, allowing good preoperative size assessment as well as assessment of invasion of the vagina, parametria, pelvic wall, bladder or rectum (Figure 15.18).

Nabothian cysts

Although there is no need to diagnose these cysts by MRI, they are a common finding and should not be confused with other lesions. These cysts are identified as well-defined round cervical masses that are

isointense on T1-weighted images and high in signal intensity on T2-weighted images (Figure 15.19)[24].

Endometrium

Endometrial carcinoma

Although MRI demonstrates abnormalities of the endometrium, the findings are non-specific. Early endometrial carcinoma (Figure 15.20) and endometrial hyperplasia have a similar appearance (endometrial thickness > 4 mm in postmenopausal women), and a histological diagnosis is required[25]. MRI has been successfully used in some centers to predict the invasion of myometrium and for local staging in cases of known endometrial carcinoma. Loss of the junctional zone can be predictive of invasion into the underlying myometrium. MRI is 85% accurate in predicting the depth of such invasion[26]. Preoperative MRI has been shown in one

Figure 15.19 Nabothian cysts of the cervix. Sagittal T2-weighted MRI through the uterus and cervix showing two well-defined, high-signal-intensity, round nabothian cysts (arrows) in the cervix

Figure 15.20 Endometrial cancer. Stage I disease. (a) A sagittal T2-weighted MRI demonstrates a large heterogeneous mass (M) distending the endometrial canal but not extending beyond the myometrium. The hypointense junctional zone, while thinned, is intact (arrows). Note a small hypointense leiomyoma (open arrow) within the myometrium, just superior to the bladder (B). (b) A corresponding sagittal T1-weighted fat-saturated post-gadolinium MRI demonstrates the mass (M) to enhance heterogeneously and to a far lesser degree than the surrounding normal myometrium

study to decrease the incidence of lymph node dissections, reducing overall costs[27].

Endometrial polyp

In one study, the detection of endometrial polyps was found to be 79% with MRI[28]. However, benign polyps cannot be reliably distinguished from polypoid endometrial cancer. Submucosal leiomyomas are differentiated by their characteristic low signal intensity on T1- and T2-weighted images (Figure 15.21).

Adnexa

Adnexal cystic masses

Adnexal masses are identified on MRI with a 95% sensitivity (Figure 15.22)[29]. The appearance of many adnexal masses is non-specific and, as with ultrasound, malignant masses cannot be completely distinguished from benign. However, several entities, including dermoid cysts, most endometriomas, pedunculated leiomyomas, hydrosalpinx and ovarian fibromas, can have specific findings and are characterized by MRI[9]. Follicular, corpus luteal and simple cysts all appear as high-signal, homogeneous, well-defined masses with no identifiable wall. Ovarian carcinomas tend to be larger with demonstrable solid components. The application of MRI in pelvic masses

Figure 15.21 Endometrial polyp and leiomyomas. (a) Midline sagittal T2-weighted MRI demonstrates two typical low-signal-intensity intramural leiomyomas (L); the larger is fundal and the second is in the posterior wall. Centrally located is a high-signal-intensity submucosal mass (arrow), just above the endocervical canal (long arrow). (b) Sagittal T1-weighted fat-saturated post-gadolinium image shows that the leiomyomas (L) and the submucosal mass (arrow) enhance. The high signal intensity on the T2-weighted image is atypical for a leiomyoma and, given its location, endometrial polyp and carcinoma must be considered in the differential diagnosis. This was a benign polyp on histology

Figure 15.22 Cystic adnexal mass: ovarian cystadenoma. (a) An axial T2-weighted MRI demonstrates a small high-signal-intensity cystic left ovarian mass (M), with no internal septations and a small focus of focal nodular wall thickening (arrow). The uterus (curved arrow) is seen anterior and medial to the mass; note the high-signal normal endometrium in its center (arrowhead). (b) A sagittal T1-weighted fat-saturated post-gadolinium MR image demonstrates no enhancement in the vast majority of this cystic lesion, aside from an enhancing area of mild focal wall thickening present superiorly (arrow)

goes beyond lesion detection and characterization to include disease staging[30].

Endometrioma

Endometriomas appear typically as round or oval well-defined adnexal masses with a thick low-signal wall and a central high signal on T1-weighted sequences (Figure 15.23). When this pattern is found, MRI is between 91 and 98% specific in making the diagnosis[9]. Lipid within a cystic teratoma may have a similar appearance on standard

158

Figure 15.23 Bilateral endometriomas. Three images of a single patient are presented. (a) An axial T2-weighted image demonstrates bilateral well-defined masses (M) on each side of the uterus (arrow), which are of low signal intensity. (b) An axial T1-weighted image demonstrates both masses (M) to be high in signal. The high signal could represent blood products in an endometrioma or fat within a cystic teratoma. (c) A chemically selective fat-saturated T1-weighted image shows the masses (M) to remain high in signal while the fat in the bone marrow and subcutaneous tissues is suppressed and appears dark. This indicates that the lesions are endometriomas

sequences; for this reason, special fat-suppression sequences are used to differentiate these lesions.

Cystic teratoma (dermoid)

Using standard as well as fat-suppressing imaging sequences, lipid can be identified with confidence (Figure 15.24). The presence of lipid in an adnexal mass identifies it, for practical purposes, as a dermoid; MRI is highly specific in making this diagnosis[9].

CONCLUSIONS

Although other methods of evaluating the female pelvis, including laparoscopy, hysteroscopy, colposcopy and ultrasonography, are often superior in both sensitivity and specificity to either CT or MRI, it is still incumbent on the gynecologist to understand these techniques. There are several indications in which CT and MRI are superior to other modalities. In addition, the global view provided by these modalities can be very helpful in confusing clinical settings. Finally, many patients undergo these studies for other reasons and are subsequently referred to the gynecologist because of the abnormalities of the female genital tract that are revealed. Understanding the value and limitations of the initial modality will enable the practitioner to proceed logically with further studies or treatment.

Figure 15.24 Ovarian dermoid. Three images of a single patient are presented. (a) An axial T2-weighted image demonstrates a well-defined, high-signal-intensity mass (arrow) to the right of the uterus. The high signal could be due to fat in a cystic teratoma or, as in Figure 15.23, hemorrhage in an endometrioma. (b) An axial T1-weighted image demonstrates the mass (arrow) to be high in signal, similar to fat. (c) A chemically selective fat-saturated T1-weighted image shows the mass (arrow) to be suppressed along with the fat in the bone marrow and subcutaneous tissues. This indicates that the lesion has lipid content and, therefore, represents an ovarian dermoid. If this were an endometrioma, it would have remained high in signal

REFERENCES

1. Buy JN, Ghossain MA, Moss AA, *et al.* Cystic teratoma of the ovary: CT detection. *Radiology* 1989;171:697–701

2. Kawamoto S, Urban BA, Fishman EK. CT of epithelial ovarian tumors. *Radiographics* 1999;19:S85–S102

3. Sam JW, Jacobs JE, Birnbaum BA. Spectrum of CT findings in acute pyogenic pelvic inflammatory disease. *Radiographics* 2002;22:1327–34

4. Raptopoulos V, Katsou G, Rosen MP, *et al.* Acute appendicitis: effect of increased use of CT on selecting patients earlier. *Radiology* 2003;226:521–6

5. Raman SS, Lu DS, Kadell BM, *et al.* Accuracy of nonfocused helical CT for the diagnosis of acute appendicitis: a 5-year review. *Am J Roentgenol* 2002;178:1319–25

6. Einstein DM, Singer AA, Chilcote WA, Desai RK. Abdominal lymphadenopathy: spectrum of CT findings. *Radiographics* 1991;11:457–72

7. Brown HK, Stoll BS, Nicosia SV, *et al.* Uterine junctional zone: correlation of histological findings and MR imaging. *Radiology* 1991;179:409–13

8. Olson M, Posniak H, Tempany CM, *et al.* MR imaging of the female pelvic region. *Radiographics* 1992;12:445–65

9. Outwater EK, Dunton CJ. Imaging of the ovary and adnexa: clinical issues and applications of MR imaging. *Radiology* 1995; 194:1–18

10. Schwartz LB, Panagaes E, Lange R, *et al.* Female pelvis: impact of MR imaging on treatment decisions and net cost analysis. *Radiology* 1994;192:55–60

11. Hricak H, Yu KK. Radiology in invasive cervical cancer. *Am J Roentgenol* 1996; 167:1101–8

12. Pellerito JS, McCarthy SM, Doyle MB, *et al.* Diagnosis of uterine anomalies: relative accuracy of MR imaging, endovaginal sonography and hysterosalpingography. *Radiology* 1992;183:795–800

13. Doyle MB. Magnetic resonance imaging in müllerian fusion defects. *J Reprod Med* 1992;37:33–8

14. Dueholm M, Lundorf E, Hansen ES, *et al.* Accuracy of magnetic resonance imaging and transvaginal ultrasonography in the diagnosis, mapping and measurement of uterine leiomyomas. *Am J Obstet Gynecol* 2002;186:409–15

15. Imaoka I, Wada A, Matsuo M, *et al.* MR Imaging of disorders associated with female infertility: use in diagnosis, treatment and management. *Radiographics* 2003;23:1401–21

16. Yamashita Y, Torashima M, Takahashi M, *et al.* Hyperintense uterine leiomyoma at T2-weighted MR imaging: Differentiation with dynamic enhanced MR imaging and clinical implications. *Radiology* 1993;189:721–5

17. Omary RA, Vasireddy S, Chrisman HB, *et al.* The effect of pelvic MR imaging on the diagnosis and treatment of women with presumed symptomatic uterine fibroids. *J Vasc Interv Radiol* 2002;13:1149–53

18. Byun JY, Kim SE, Choi BG, *et al.* Diffuse and focal adenomyosis: MR imaging findings. *Radiographics* 1999;19:S161–S170

19. Outwater EK, Siegelman ES, Deerlin VV. Adenomyosis: current concepts and imaging considerations. *Am J Roentgenol* 1998;170: 437–41

20. Reinhold C, McCarthy S, Bret PM, *et al.* Diffuse adenomyosis: comparison of endovaginal US and MR imaging with histopathologic correlation. *Radiology* 1996;199:151–8

21. Togashi K, Ozasa I, Konishi I, *et al.* Enlarged uterus: differentiation between adenomyosis and leiomyoma with MR imaging. *Radiology* 1989;171:531–54

22. Hricak H, Powell CB, Yu KK, *et al.* Invasive cervical carcinoma: role of MR imaging in pre-treatment work-up – cost minimization and diagnostic efficacy analysis. *Radiology* 1996;198:403–9

23. Kaur H, Silverman PM, Iyer RB, *et al.* Diagnosis, staging and surveillance of cervical carcinoma. *Am J Roentgenol* 2003; 180:1621–32

24. Okamoto Y, Tanaka YO, Nishida M, *et al.* MR imaging of the uterine cervix: imaging–pathologic correlation. *Radiographics* 2003;23:425–45

25. Brown JJ, Thurnher S, Hricak H. MR imaging of the uterus: low-signal-intensity abnormalities of the endometrium and endometrial cavity. *Magn Reson Imaging* 1990;8:309–13

26. Yamshita Y, Harada M, Sawada T, *et al.* Normal uterus and FIGO stage I endometrial carcinoma: dynamic gadolinium-enhanced MR imaging. *Radiology* 1993;186:495–501

27. Hardesty LA, Sumkin JH, Nath ME, *et al.* Use of preoperative MR imaging in the management of endometrial carcinoma: cost analysis. *Radiology* 2000;215:45–9

28. Hricak H, Finck S, Honda G, Goranson H. MR imaging in the evaluation of benign uterine masses: value of gadopentetate dimeglumine-enhanced T1-weighted images. *Am J Roentgenol* 1992;158:1043–50

29. Stevens SK, Hricak H, Stern JL. Ovarian lesions: detection and characterization with gadolinium-enhanced MR imaging at 1.5T. *Radiology* 1991;181:481–8

30. Szklaruk J, Tamm EP, Choi H, *et al.* MR imaging of common and uncommon large pelvic masses. *Radiographics* 2003;23:403–24

16

Uterine pathology

Debra S. Heller

The pathology laboratory often receives specimens obtained during hysteroscopy and is able to confirm the hysteroscopic impression. Hysteroscopic visualization is particularly helpful in identifying focal rather than diffuse lesions (Figure 16.1). Although many of these specimens are identical in appearance to those obtained by other operative modalities, some specimens are received in fragments or with cautery artifact after operative hysteroscopic resection, thereby occasionally hampering interpretation. The various types of specimens received by the pathology laboratory from hysteroscopic procedures are listed in Table 16.1.

ABNORMAL UTERINE BLEEDING

Abnormal uterine bleeding may occur under a variety of conditions. After eliminating non-uterine causes such as systemic disease or non-genital bleeding, and ruling out pregnancy-related bleeding, uterine bleeding may be classified as either organic or dysfunctional. Organic causes of bleeding are those associated with intrinsic uterine pathology, such as a polyp or submucous leiomyoma. Dysfunctional uterine bleeding (DUB) is secondary to an imbalance of the hormonal milieu. The endometrium in cases of DUB may appear

Figure 16.1 Hysterectomy specimen showing focal thickening of the endometrium

completely normal or may show a variety of patterns, both non-secretory and secretory.

MENSTRUAL CYCLE

Endometrial samples obtained during an infertility work-up as well as in some cases of dysfunctional bleeding may be completely normal on histology. In these cases, the clinical history is important in determining whether the specimen is out of phase. Luteal phase defects, defined as a > 2-day discrepancy in clinical and histolog-

Table 16.1 Pathology specimens from hysteroscopic procedures

Endometrium
    history of abnormal bleeding
    infertility work-up
    abnormal transvaginal ultrasound
    abnormal Papanicolaou smear
    follow-up after hyperplasia
    endometrial polyps
    endometrial carcinoma
Retained IUD/foreign bodies
Retained products of conception/placental polyps
Endocervical polyps
Uterine septa/synechiae
Submucous smooth muscle neoplasms
Adenomyosis

ical dating, may be seen in some cases of infertility and DUB, but also occur in completely asymptomatic fertile women.

During the first half of the menstrual cycle, under the stimulus of estrogen, the endometrium becomes taller, with increased gland complexity and mitotic activity. Proliferative endometrium cannot be dated, but can be divided into early, mid- and late proliferative phases by the morphology. Early proliferative endometrium (cycle days 1–4) is characterized by simple straight glands, which appear small and round on histological section. Mitotic activity is present in both glands and stroma (Figure 16.2). During the mid-proliferative phase (cycle days 5–9), gland complexity and mitotic activity both increase, the endometrium becomes taller and stromal edema may be seen (Figure 16.3). Late proliferative endometrium (cycle days 10–14) is taller than early and mid-proliferative endometrium, and shows maximum mitotic activity. The glands are more complex in architecture, and the edema seen in the mid-proliferative phase is absent (Figure 16.4). In all phases of proliferative endometrium, the glandular epithelium is pseudostratified, thereby distinguishing it from the single layer of secretory endometrium.

Secretory endometrium can be reliably dated on a daily basis, as first described by Noyes and colleagues[1]. Secretory endometrium can also be divided into early (cycle days 15–19), mid- (cycle days 20–24) and late (cycle days 25–28). It was originally thought that, whereas the proliferative phase of the cycle was variable, the secretory phase was fixed at 14 days. This has proved to be not the case and normally fertile women can have variable cycles[2]. For this reason, it is better not to diagnose a luteal phase defect unless the endometrium is more than 2 days out of phase in more than one cycle.

During the early secretory phase, it is not possible to determine histologically whether or not ovulation has occurred until cycle day 17. Day-15 endometrium may show a few subnuclear vacuoles and up to 50% of glands may show subnuclear vacuolization on day 16, but this may be seen secondary to estrogenic stimulation alone

Figure 16.2 Early proliferative endometrium showing small tubular glands. Glandular epithelium is pseudostratified and mitotically active (hematoxylin and eosin, H&E)

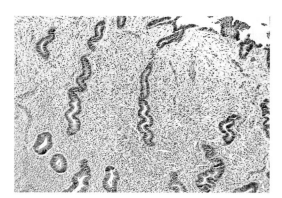

Figure 16.3 Mid-proliferative endometrium shows increased gland complexity and an edematous stroma (H&E)

Figure 16.4 Late proliferative endometrium showing markedly increased gland tortuosity. Peak glandular and stromal mitotic activity occurs at this time (H&E)

Figure 16.5 Day-17 secretory endometrium showing uniform subnuclear vacuoles (H&E)

in the absence of progesterone; mitotic activity is still abundant. The morphology of day-17 endometrium (Figure 16.5) allows a reliable determination that ovulation has occurred. The glands show uniform subnuclear vacuolization and give the appearance of piano keys. At day 17, there is only a single layer of glandular epithelium and mitotic activity is minimal. As the early secretory phase progresses, the vacuoles migrate to a supranuclear location,

with peak secretion on day 20. It is often difficult to assign an exact day to endometrium in the day 19–21 range (Figure 16.6), but peak stromal edema is seen on day 22 (Figure 16.7) and spiral arterioles become prominent on day 23 (Figure 16.8). Predecidual cuffing is present around the spiral arterioles and spreads outwards during the late secretory period. There is increased cuffing on day 24, the presence of predecidua under the surface by day 25 and complete stromal predecidualization by day 27 (Figure 16.9).

Figure 16.6 Day-19–21 secretory endometrium in low- (a) and high- (b) power views showing both subnuclear and supranuclear vacuoles. The glandular epithelium is single-layered and lacks mitotic activity (H&E)

Figure 16.7 Day-22 secretory endometrium shows peak stromal edema (H & E)

Breakdown and menses begin on day 28. Menstrual endometrium is characterized by gland–stroma dissociation, stromal clumping, fibrin thrombi in vessels and nuclear 'dust' (Figure 16.10).

ATROPHY

Postmenopausal endometrium may exhibit one of two common atrophic patterns: atrophy may be diffuse, with a thin endometrium and inactive glands (Figure 16.11); or it may occur in another common pattern,

Figure 16.8 Day-23 secretory endometrium in low- (a) and high- (b) power views shows prominent spiral arterioles with perivascular cuffing by predecidua (H&E)

Figure 16.9 Low- (a) and high- (b) power views of day-27 secretory endometrium show complete prede-cidualization of the stroma (H&E)

Figure 16.10 Menstrual endometrium shows breakdown and stromal clumping. Only from early menstrual endometrium is it possible to determine whether ovulation has occurred. In this example, secretory changes are still recognizable (H&E)

Figure 16.11 Atrophic endometrium is often seen in specimens from postmenopausal women; only superficial strips of inactive glandular epithelium are seen here (H&E)

cystic atrophy, with widely dilated glands (Figure 16.12). This latter pattern may be distinguished from hyperplasia by the flat epithelium in the cystic glands, which are devoid of mitotic activity.

IATROGENIC HORMONAL EFFECTS

Endometrium stimulated by exogenous hormone therapy shows a pattern that reflects both the medication, dose and duration as well as the underlying hormon-

al milieu of the patient. This is particularly evident in postmenopausal women receiving estrogen/progesterone replacement therapy, when the endometrium may appear atrophic, proliferative, secretory or irregular, with mixed proliferative and secretory features (Figure 16.13). If estrogen stimulation is excessive, hyperplastic and malignant patterns may also be seen.

Prolonged oral contraception as well as progestational therapy for abnormal bleeding results in endometrium with small atrophic glands and decidualized

Figure 16.12 Cystic atrophy is characterized by cystically dilated glands lined by flattened inactive epithelium (H&E)

Figure 16.13 Hormone replacement therapy can result in an endometrium showing both proliferative and secretory features, as seen here (H&E)

Figure 16.14 Progesterone therapy can result in a picture of inactive glands in a decidualized stroma (H&E)

Figure 16.15 Gonadotropin-releasing hormone (GnRH) agonist therapy may result in an atrophic endometrium (H&E)

stroma (Figure 16.14). Therapy with gonadotropin-releasing hormone (GnRH) agonists creates an artificial menopause with an atrophic endometrium (Figure 16.15). Tamoxifen, which exerts an antiestrogenic effect on breast carcinoma, has a weak estrogenic effect on the postmenopausal uterus. In addition to endometrial hyperplasia and carcinoma, endometrial and endocervical polyps, and growth of adenomyosis, endometriosis and leiomyomas have been described. Endometrial polyps arising after tamoxifen therapy are often large with a

densely fibrotic stroma and cystically dilated glands[3] (Figure 16.16).

DYSFUNCTIONAL UTERINE BLEEDING

Dysfunctional uterine bleeding (DUB), defined as bleeding in the absence of systemic disease, pregnancy or intrauterine lesion, is due to hormonal imbalance. Both non-secretory and secretory patterns may be seen[4]. The most common cause of DUB is anovulation. Anovulatory endometrium

Figure 16.16 Endometrial polyps from patients taking tamoxifen are often large, with cystically dilated glands and a densely fibrous stroma (H&E)

Figure 16.17 Anovulatory menstrual endometrium exhibiting breakdown on a background of disordered proliferation (see Figure 16.18; H&E)

may appear as normal proliferative, proliferative with breakdown, disordered proliferative or even as hyperplasia/carcinoma in the presence of continued unopposed estrogen stimulation. Disordered proliferation (Figures 16.17, 16.18) is c haracterized by scattered, cystically dilated, glands in a proliferative background with no increase in the gland : stroma ratio, and is not considered hyperplastic. Endometrial ablation may be performed in cases of recurrent DUB, but does not result in a specimen for pathological evaluation. A more recent technique, endomyometrial resection[5], removes the entire endometrium in strips with myometrium (Figure 16.19).

Figure 16.18 Disordered proliferation of the endometrium in anovulatory cycles may show a few cystically dilated glands mixed with a proliferative pattern. The gland : stroma ratio is not increased; the picture is not considered severe enough to be classified as hyperplasia (H&E)

ENDOMETRIAL POLYPS

The ideal endometrial polyp, from a pathologist's point of view, is intact with an endometrial epithelial lining on three sides, and a prominent stalk with thick-walled vessels. Often, polyps are removed in fragments, and the irregular, stellate, non-secretory glands and fibrotic stroma

have to be relied upon to make the diagnosis (Figure 16.20).

ENDOMETRIAL HYPERPLASIA

Endometrial hyperplasia has numerous and often confusing classification systems. The most common system in current use categorizes the hyperplasias by both architecture

Figure 16.19 Endomyometrial resection: (a) view through a Storz (Culver City, CA) resectoscope, 25-Fr diameter with a 30° foreoblique lens, shows resection of an endomyometrial cardinal strip from the anterior uterine wall; (b) the resected endomyometrial strips (a) and (b), courtesy of Morris Wortman, MD); (c) low-power view of a strip removed by resection shows cautery artifact (H&E)

Figure 16.20 (a) A pedunculated endometrial polyp is seen arising from the uterine cavity. (b) Low- (b) and higher- (c) power views of an endometrial polyp showing irregular stellate glands and thick vessels in the stalk (H&E)

Figure 16.21 Simple hyperplasia shows mild glandular crowding (H&E)

Figure 16.22 Complex hyperplasia shows increased glandular crowding (H&E)

Figure 16.23 Low- (left) and higher- (right) power views of atypical hyperplasia (complex hyperplasia with atypia) show marked glandular crowding and nuclear atypia. The enlarged round nuclei show margination of the chromatin and prominent nucleoli (lower; H&E)

and presence or absence of nuclear atypia[6]. Glandular architecture may be either simple or complex. Simple hyperplasia (Figure 16.21) consists of a minimal-to-mild increase in the gland : stroma ratio with cystic dilatation and occasional outpouching of glands. Complex hyperplasia is used to describe more severe degrees of glandular crowding which are nevertheless insufficient to be deemed carcinoma (Figure 16.22). Atypia describes the presence of atypical glandular epithelial nuclei. Instead of the usual oval nuclei, atypical nuclei are larger and rounder, with clumping and margination of the chromatin (Figure 16.23).

There are four possible patterns of hyperplasia by this classification: simple (without atypia); simple (with atypia); complex (without atypia); and complex (with atypia). Simple hyperplasia is rarely atypical and, thus, for purposes of simplification, the terminology often consists of 'simple', 'complex' or 'atypical' hyperplasia. Atypical hyperplasia is identical to complex hyperplasia with atypia, and simple or complex hyperplasia denotes no atypia if not mentioned. The importance of this classification

Table 16.2 Endometrial carcinoma: most common histological types

Endometrioid or the usual adenocarcinoma, and variants
Endometrial adenocarcinoma with squamous differentiation
Mucinous adenocarcinoma
Clear cell adenocarcinoma
Serous carcinoma
Mixed cell type carcinoma
Undifferentiated carcinoma

Figure 16.24 Endometrial adenocarcinoma: (a) well-differentiated (grade 1) and (b) poorly differentiated (grade 3), with squamous differentiation (H&E)

rests in its predictive nature. Only atypical hyperplasia has a high likelihood of being associated with either concomitant (unsampled) carcinoma or the development of carcinoma. In the study by Kurman and co-workers[6], 23% of all patients with either type of atypical hyperplasia (29% of those with complex hyperplasia with atypia) progressed to carcinoma. Knowledge of the risk of malignancy allows planning for treatment.

ENDOMETRIAL CARCINOMA

There are several different histological subtypes of endometrial carcinoma (Table 16.2). The most prevalent is endometrioid or the usual adenocarcinoma. In the past, squamous epithelium within an endometrial adenocarcinoma led to a diagnosis of adenoacanthoma if benign in appearance, and adenosquamous carcinoma if histologically malignant. As the prognosis rests predominantly on the grade of the glandular component[7], these tumors are now graded on that component with mention of squamous differentiation (Figure 16.24). For example, a diagnosis might read grade 2 adenocarcinoma of the endometrium with squamous differentiation'. Two of the histological types – serous (Figure 16.25) and clear cell adenocarcinoma (Figure 16.26) – are significant for carrying a poorer prognosis than do the other types of endometrial cancer.

The current International Federation of Gynecologists and Obstetricians (FIGO) staging of endometrial carcinoma is based on surgical and pathological findings (Table 16.3). For early-stage tumors, the decision whether to perform lymph node sampling

Table 16.3 FIGO staging of endometrial carcinoma[8]

Stage Ia G123	Tumor limited to endometrium
Stage Ib G123	Invasion to less than one-half the myometrium
Stage Ic G123	Invasion to half or more of the myometrium
Stage IIa G123	Endocervical glandular involvement only
Stage IIb G123	Cervical stromal invasion
Stage IIIa G123	Tumor invades serosa/adnexa and/or positive peritoneal cytology
Stage IIIb G123	Vaginal metastases
Stage IIIc G123	Metastases to pelvic and/or para-aortic lymph nodes
Stage IVa G123	Tumor invasion of bladder and/or bowel mucosa
Stage IVb	Distant metastases

G123, grades 1, 2 or 3

Figure 16.25 Serous carcinoma of the endometrium is histologically similar to ovarian papillary serous cystadenocarcinoma (H&E)

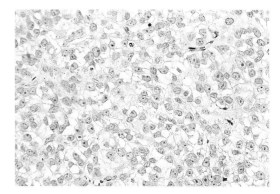

Figure 16.26 Clear cell adenocarcinoma of the endometrium (H&E)

at the time of hysterectomy often depends upon the tumor grade and depth of myometrial invasion. The grade used in this decision is often that assigned at initial sampling[9]. Endometrioid adenocarcinoma of the endometrium is graded in the FIGO system predominantly according to the architecture: grade 1 is no more than 5% solid; grade 2 is 6–50% solid; and grade 3 is over 50% solid (Figures 16.27–16.29) The tumor is upgraded by one grade for significant nuclear atypia. Caveats include not interpreting large areas of squamous meta-

Figure 16.27 Grade 1 endometrial adenocarcinoma shows back-to-back glands without intervening stroma (H&E)

Figure 16.28 Grade 2 endometrial adenocarcinoma shows a mixture of glandular and solid areas (H&E)

Figure 16.29 Grade 3 endometrial adenocarcinoma is predominantly solid (H&E)

plasia as solid adenocarcinoma. Because of their more aggressive behavior, clear cell and serous tumors are generally considered to be grade 3.

Although not commonly used in staging endometrial carcinoma, hysteroscopy may assist in detecting lesions involving the cervix as well as in pinpointing the site of initial sampling.

Uterine septa/adhesions

A pathology specimen is occasionally received after hysteroscopic metroplasty or after lysis of adhesions in a patient with Asherman's syndrome. Fragments of fibromuscular tissue, often with cautery artifact, may be seen (Figure 16.30).

MYOMETRIAL LESIONS

Submucous leiomyoma

Submucous leiomyomas may be detected, and sometimes resected, hysteroscopically. They may be removed whole, particularly if pedunculated (Figure 16.31) but, if resected

in pieces, may be difficult to distinguish from normal myometrium (Figure 16.32).

Leiomyosarcoma

Occasionally, leiomyosarcomas are detected or suspected from tissue removed hysteroscopically. The amount of tissue may be insufficient for a definitive diagnosis, which depends upon evaluating for the presence of coagulative necrosis as well as the number of mitoses per ten high-power fields and the presence or absence of atypia[10] (Figure 16.33).

Adenomyosis

Adenomyosis, consisting of both endometrial glands and stroma within the myometrium, can occasionally be diagnosed on a hysteroscopically obtained specimen (Figure 16.34).

Pregnancy and foreign bodies

Hysteroscopy may occasionally detect a placental polyp or retained products of

174

Figure 16.30 (a) Septate uterus with leiomyomas. (b) Uterine septum after hysteroscopic resection consists of fibrous tissue and endometrial fragments (H&E)

Figure 16.31 (a) Uterus with intramural and subserosal leiomyomas. (d) Submucous leiomyoma shows clearly the contour of the leiomyoma. Note the pressure atrophy of the endometrium (H&E)

175

Figure 16.32 Submucous leiomyoma fragment, removed during endomyometrial resection, shows interlacing muscle bundles that are suggestive, but not diagnostic, of leiomyoma (courtesy of Morris Wortman, MD; H&E)

Figure 16.34 Adenomyosis consists of endometrial glands and stroma within myometrium (courtesy of Morris Wortman, MD; H&E)

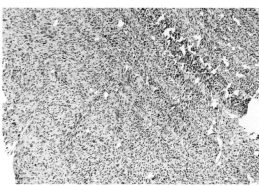

Figure 16.33 This specimen, removed during a hysteroscopic procedure, was highly suggestive of a leiomyosarcoma. This diagnosis was confirmed at hysterectomy (H&E)

conception (Figure 16.35). The most commonly detected intrauterine foreign body is an intrauterine device (IUD), which may be difficult to remove owing to retraction of the 'tail' or being imbedded in the myometrium (Figure 16.36). Removal of bone fragments[11] probably due to prior intrauterine gestation and retrieval of laminaria fragments[12] have been described.

Figure 16.35 Placental polyp shows 'ghost' chorionic villi (H&E)

Figure 16.36 Retained IUD with adhesion

REFERENCES

1. Noyes RW, Hertig AT, Rock J. Dating the endometrial biopsy. *Fertil Steril* 1950;1:3–25

2. Langren BM, Unden AL, Diczfalusy E. Hormonal profile of the cycle in 68 normally menstruating women. *Acta Endocrinol Copenh* 1980;94:89–98

3. Nuovo MA, Nuovo GJ, McCaffrey R, *et al.* Endometrial polyps in postmenopausal patients receiving tamoxifen. *Int J Gynecol Pathol* 1989;8:125–31

4. Heller D. *The Endometrium: A Clinicopathologic Approach.* New York: Igaku-Shoin Medical Publishers, 1994:76–80

5. Wortman M, Daggett A. Hysteroscopic endomyometrial resection: a new technique for the treatment of menorrhagia. *Obstet Gynecol* 1994;83:295–8

6. Kurman RJ, Kaminsky PF, Norris HJ. The behavior of endometrial hyperplasia: a long-term study of 'untreated' hyperplasia in 170 patients. *Cancer* 1985;56:403–12

7. Zaino RJ, Kurman RJ. Squamous differentiation in carcinoma of the endometrium: a critical appraisal of adenoacanthoma and adenosquamous carcinoma. *Semin Diagn Pathol* 1988;5:154–71

8. Green FL, ed. *AJCC Cancer Staging Manual,* 6th edn. New York: Springer-Verlag, 2002

9. Heller D, Drosinos S, Westhoff C. Accuracy of tumor grade assigned at initial endometrial sampling [Letter]. *Int J Gynecol Obstet* 1994;47:301–2

10. Bell SW, Kempson RL, Hendrickson MR. Problematic uterine smooth muscle neoplasms. A clinicopathologic study of 213 cases. *Am J Surg Pathol* 1994;18:535-58.

11. Marcus SF, Bhattacharya J, Williams G, *et al.* Endometrial ossification: a cause of secondary infertility. *Am J Obstet Gynecol* 1994;170:1381–3

12. Borgatta L, Barad D. Prolonged retention of laminaria fragments: an unusual complication of laminaria usage. *Obstet Gynecol* 1991;78:988–90

Epilogue

Hysteroscopy has achieved its proper place in modern gynecology. The early problems associated with its performance have been solved with new instrumentation and the safe use of CO_2 gas and/or low-viscosity fluids to distend the uterine cavity with simple and effective methods of delivery. Light sources have been improved and miniature cameras with excellent resolution introduced, adding to the armamentarium and safety of the technique. Video hysteroscopy is now a routine method of evaluation and treatment. Office hysteroscopy has been made possible with simpler instrumentation and endoscopes that do not require cervical dilatation, thereby reducing patient inconvenience and discomfort, saving physician time and inconvenience, and eliminating the bureaucracy entailed with the use of ambulatory surgical centers or operating suites. The diagnostic applications of hysteroscopy are well-defined, enabling evaluation not only of structural abnormalities such as myomas, polyps, anatomical anomalies and pathological scars that distort the uterine cavity, but also the different changes that the endometrium may undergo, whether benign, premalignant and/or malignant.

The therapeutic applications of hysteroscopy have expanded and are also well-defined. The uterine septum can be treated transcervically, thereby supplanting abdominal metroplasty; submucous leiomyomas can be safely resected without the need for a laparotomy; and intrauterine adhesions can be divided with greater precision to provide an improved reproductive outcome compared with the previous blind or more invasive methods of treatment. Tubal cannulation for cornual occlusion is now the first step in the evaluation and treatment, allowing the selection of only those patients with fibrotic occlusions who will benefit most from microsurgical resection and anastomosis or *in vitro* fertilization and embryo transfer. Endometrial ablation is a viable alternative to hysterectomy for women with dysfunctional uterine bleeding that is unresponsive to hormonal treatment. Tubal sterilization, using microinserts deployed by hysteroscopy, is now performed in the clinical setting.

Finally, new and promising hysteroscopic applications are on the horizon. Technological improvements and adaptation of various techniques may eventually prove beneficial for the use of hysteroscopy and include embryoscopy, direct visual delivery of gametes, zygotes or embryos into the uterine cavity, and a practical method of observing and evaluating the intratubal epithelium from the uterine side.

Hysteroscopy has a well-earned place in gynecology today and should be used in patients who may benefit from intrauterine visualization.

Index